HOMEOPATHY

OPTIMA

ALTERNATIVE HEALTH

HOMEOPATHY

DR NELSON BRUNTON

ILLUSTRATED BY SHAUN WILLIAMS

An OPTIMA book

First published in 1989 by
Macdonald Optima
This edition published by Optima in 1992

© Dr Nelson Brunton 1989

British Library Cataloguing in Publication Data
Brunton, Nelson
Homeopathy.—(Alternative health series).
1. Medicine. Homeopathy
I. Title   II. Series
615.5′32

ISBN 0-356-20993-8

Photoset in Century Schoolbook by
Leaper & Gard Ltd, Bristol, England
Printed in England by Clays Ltd, St Ives plc

Optima Books
A Division of
Little, Brown and Company (UK) Limited
165 Great Dover Street
London SE1 4YA

DEDICATION

I would like to dedicate this book to my parents who educated me when times were hard, my wife Patricia who was very patient and understanding with me while I wrote this book and, last but not least, my two daughters Shiene and Rachel who have given me great inspiration.

CONTENTS

ACKNOWLEDGEMENTS

'*Ye who has good friends is truly wealthy.*' I would like to take the opportunity to thank all those who helped me in the writing of this book: my wife Patricia who was kept awake reading to me till late into the night; Liz Deakin who took shorthand and did most of the typing; Roy Borley who spent many hours making cross-references for me; Doreen Boulter who has been a true critic, helping to improve the quality of the writing and correcting the manuscript. Special thanks are also due to my very great friends and colleagues Dr Michael Nightingale, without whose help this book would never have been written, and Professor Dr Anton Jayasuriya, for inviting me to hear his inspiring lectures during my many teaching visits to the Colombo South Government General Hospital, Sri Lanka, which were sponsored and promoted by Medicina Alternativa.

1.
WHAT IS HOMEOPATHY?

Allopathy (orthodox medicine) views the human body as being rather like a machine, parts of which can go wrong or wear out and they have to be repaired or replaced. The system is based on the principle of treating diseases according to the laws of opposites: heat with cold, germs with antibiotics, constipation with laxatives, coughing with suppressant drugs, inflammation with anti-inflammatory drugs and so on.

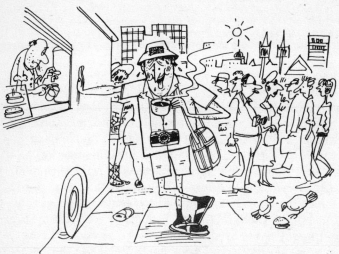

WE ARE ALL AWARE OF THE REFRESHING EFFECTS OF A HOT CUP OF TEA ON A WARM SUMMER'S DAY...

Homeopathy, on the other hand, is based on the principle of treating like with like. Accordingly, heat cures the effects of heat (we are all aware of the refreshing effects of a hot cup of tea on a warm summer's day), purgatives help to cure diarrhoea and, since nettles cause a burning itch, they will cure nettle-rash.

The allopathic approach is to identify and treat specific diseases caused by viruses, germs and bacteria which enter the body and lower its resistance. When these microscopic organisms increase and multiply and the body weakens, symptoms appear to inform us of what is going wrong within. Allopathic medicines are designed to act against these symptoms.

In homeopathy, however, it is the *patient* who is treated, *not* the disease. (If homeopaths use the names of diseases at all, it is merely to help communicate with a patient who has been indoctrinated into that way of thinking.) Homeopathic remedies work to re-establish the flow of the body's 'vital force' so that it regains its natural balance, thus eliminating symptoms and preventing them in the future.

SAMUEL HAHNEMANN AND HOMEOPATHY

Homeopathy in its classic form was developed by the German doctor Christian Samuel Hahnemann, who was born on 10 April 1755 in Meissen (now in East Germany). His father, a porcelain painter, encouraged the young Samuel to think for himself by giving him problems to solve. This slightly unusual upbringing undoubtedly helped Hahnemann's development as an original thinker.

At the age of 20, he began studying medicine at Leipzig University, supporting himself by teaching languages and translating. After graduating, he had the good fortune to be apprenticed to Freiherr von Quarin, physician to the Empress of Austria and principal physician at the Hospital of the Brothers of Charity. Hahnemann said later that he owed all his skills as a physician to the experience he gained with Dr von Quarin.

After his apprenticeship, Hahnemann spent two years as family doctor in Hermannstadt, and subsequently completed his medical studies in Erlangen with a thesis on the causes and treatment of spasmodic bowel disorders. He then established a practice in Hettstadt, subsequently studying pharmacology and completing his practical training at the Mohren Pharmacy in Dessau. One attraction of the pharmacy proved to be the apothecary's step-daughter, Henrietta, whom Hahnemann married a year later. Soon after, he was appointed Medical Officer of Health at Dessau.

THE DISCOVERY OF PROVINGS

By the time his wife had given birth to five of their 11 children, Hahnemann had become disillusioned with medicine as it was then being practised and, abandoning his official post, once again took to translating in order to support his family. In 1790, while working on a pharmacology textbook by Cullin of Edinburgh, his reading led him to formulate the principles known today as homeopathy. Hahnemann found that he could not accept the explanation given for the way in which herbs (the drugs of the 18th century) were supposed to work, and he decided that the only way to discover their true action was to test them on himself. This process is now well known to all homeopaths as a *proving*.

He started with cinchona, the South American bark that is the source of quinine, and which was the primary treatment for malaria. To his surprise, he found that, when he took this, it produced in him the very symptoms of the disease which the drug was being used to cure — namely, intermittent fever, aches and pains, and loss of vital fluids causing weakness. When he stopped taking quinine, all the symptoms gradually disappeared.

Hahnemann continued to experiment, carrying out provings of many of the drugs then in current use, both on himself and on friends who had volunteered to help him. Some idea of Hahnemann's immense industry can be given by the fact that he 'proved' over 90 different drugs. These provings formed the basis of his *Materia Medica Pura*, which was first published in 1811 and became a classic textbook for all serious homeopathic practitioners.

THE LAW OF SIMILARS

Now able to predict the action of many drugs, Hahnemann devised a revolutionary system of medicine based on the principle of matching the symptoms of a patient to the symptoms produced by a proven drug. When the chosen drug, or 'remedy', was given, it helped to strengthen the flow of the body's 'vital force', enabling the body to overcome the symptoms. This 'Law of Similars' was not new — the basic idea had been known even in the time of Hippocrates — but it took the genius of Hahnemann to incorporate it into a complete system of medicine.

Shortly after his discovery, Hahnemann was able to put his theory to the test: when an epidemic of typhoid fever swept through Napoleon's army, he treated 180 cases; only one soldier died, despite the severity of the disease and the low resistance of the men. This triumph of homeopathy made Hahnemann famous.

THE LAW OF THE MINIMUM DOSE

Hahnemann then set out to find the smallest amounts that were needed for drugs to be beneficial and not produce adverse side-effects. He was probably aware of what had happened to a herbalist who had practised his art in rural Germany. On one occasion, during a widespread epidemic, the herbalist began to run out of

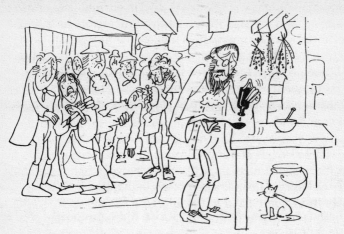

DURING A WIDESPREAD EPIDEMIC, THE HERBALIST BEGAN TO RUN OUT OF SUPPLIES...

supplies. Rather than turn people away, he began to dilute his herbal mixtures and was amazed to find that people still got better.

Hahnemann, too, was surprised when he found that the more he diluted a drug, the more potent was its healing power. This principle, which he incorporated into homeopathy, is known today as the 'Law of the Minimum Dose'.

When Hahnemann first treated his patients applying his new principle, he administered remedies in measurable doses — for example, one tenth of a gram of arsenic for the treatment of diarrhoea. These were known as 'material doses'. As time progressed, he began to use ever smaller doses, realizing that he achieved better results if he did so.

SUCCUSSION AND POTENCY

Hahnemann then found that if he were to *succuss* (or shake vigorously) his remedies each time he diluted them, this would dramatically affect their 'potency' — their therapeutic effect. Although the material substance (the amount of the actual drug) became less and less every time the process of diluting and succussion took place, the potency increased. By the time a remedy had undergone the twenty-fifth potency — in other words, the process had taken place 25 times — there was no material substance left in the dilution. However, in its place was the dynamic energy of the *vital force*, which, Hahnemann believed, animates all living things (see below).

This practice of dilution and succussion became a cornerstone of homeopathy. What seems to happen is that the substance itself is not 'potentized', but a force of vibration is imparted to the diluted substance.

When a drug is diluted to one part in ten and then succussed, it is termed a '1x' or first *decimal* potency (in Europe, this is often expressed as '1D'). When a drop of the 1x solution is similarly diluted and succussed again, it then becomes a '2x' and so on. The most commonly used decimal potency is 6x, although sometimes a 12x is used. In a 6x, the drug is present in the dilution as one part per million.

There is another scale of dilution, known as the *centesimal* potency. In this, the drug is diluted to one part in 100 each time it is diluted and succussed. The first dilution is 1c, and the lowest potency in common use in this range is 6c, which means that the drug has been diluted this way six times. Very often the 'c' is left out and only the number is used, so '200' would mean that the drug has been diluted 200 times.

An 'M' potency means that the drug has been diluted 1,000 times. Hahnemann later went on to produce remedies on this *millesimal* scale, discovering that the higher potencies helped to achieve maximum effect from the drug, with minimum side-effects, or 'aggravation' (see pages 43-4).

Any potency above 200c is said to be a 'high potency'. Generally speaking, low-potency remedies are used in first aid (see Chapter 4), or when the case is not clear or internal tissues or organs are severely damaged. When the case *is* clear and the *similimum* (the remedy that most closely matches the illness) has been selected, a high potency is used. Some practitioners use only low-potency remedies preferring the broader spectrum of activity that they offer.

ARDNT-SCHULTZ LAW

Ardnt and Schultz were two physicists who discovered that in relation to general biological activity:

- *weak* stimuli *encourage* life activity
- *medium-strength* stimuli *impede* life activity
- *strong* stimuli *stop* or *destroy* life activity.

For example, a large amount of arsenic will kill a yeast culture, a lesser amount will impede its activity, and a small amount will actually encourage the fermentation process. This is one of the fundamental laws of homeopathy.

THE VITAL FORCE

According to homeopathy, the 'vital force' is the unseen spiritual energy, or 'vital principle', that activates the body and promotes healing. This energy permeates all of nature, and without it, nothing can exist.

When the vital force is disturbed, there is disharmony, and this produces symptoms that prevent the body from functioning normally. Disease is not an entity in itself: it is the body's way of informing us that something is wrong. Symptoms are caused by the body's attempt to regain harmony and balance. The most basic upset of the vital force is where there is stagnation or accumulation of, say, body fluids; this results in pain. Where there is a deficiency in the body, there is often numbness.

Homeopathy also recognizes the paramount importance

of the mind and its interplay with the body: remedies are selected as much for the way they affect mental activity as for anything else. High-potency remedies act predominantly on the mind and spirit, and in the removal of symptoms due to miasmatic (long-standing or suppressed) effects (see below), whereas low potencies, being more material, act predominantly on the body.

The spiritual being is nourished by the principle of love. Hatred, anger and violence destroy the love within, resulting in a condition in which the vital force cannot flow in harmony with the body. Disease is often the result. The apoplectic, red-faced executive who suffers a heart attack, the brave widow who holds in her grief and develops arthritis, the assembly-line worker, under stress and with no control over his working life, who develops a peptic ulcer — all are examples of people whose vital force is suppressed and who end up with a physical manifestation of their inner imbalance.

MIASMS

Hahnemann also noticed that a remedy sometimes did not work despite the fact that it had been correctly chosen and given in the right potency. At other times, after a temporary improvement, a patient would return with a recurrence of the old symptoms or with some new ones. After many years of careful research, he found that these patients invariably had previous skin problems or even an itch, which they had tended to overlook. He concluded that these conditions were 'blocking' the action of the remedy, and he called this a *miasm*.

A miasm is the inherited effect of a disease that has been suppressed. It is the thread that runs through the history of humankind from its most distant origins to the present day. It is the omnipresent pollution of the vital force, which lies at the root of all disease. The most ancient miasm, the primary disease of all mankind, Hahnemann termed the *psora*, although he and his later followers also identified other miasms that had their origins in the serious and chronic diseases prevalent at the time: syphilis, sycosis (gonorrhoea) and tuberculosis.

It is important to realize, however, that a miasm is not the original disease but a 'residue' left by it and passed on from generation to generation. Many of today's diseases are the aftermath of these miasms.

The psora

The fundamental miasm is the psora, and without it, the others could not have developed. How then did the psora begin? Homeopaths believe that the psora exists in all thinking species, and may be seen as the result of suppressed or over-stimulated thought — we have all experienced how, if we dwell (consciously or unconsciously) on one part of the body, this frequently results in an irritation or itch in that area. It is inconceivable that such an all-pervading infection as the psora could have arisen in a being in a perfect state of health who lived in harmony with the laws of nature. Therefore, at some time or other, a distortion must have occurred in the natural order of evolution, when uncontrolled thoughts and desires interrupted the flow of

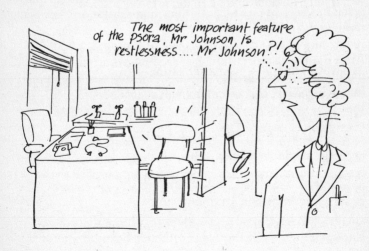

the vital force resulting in physical disharmony.

The most important feature of the psora is restlessness. Disharmony with the environment will never allow the psoric person to be satisfied with the existing state of things. Alongside this restlessness is a discreet, yet powerful reminder of guilt. The psoric will be fearful of common, harmless things such as the dark, the future or being alone when mildly under the weather. Fear of losing what one possesses is another characteristic of the psoric person, who tends to be a miserly collector of trivial things.

The psoric miasm shows itself externally as skin problems, mainly an itchy, dry and cracked skin. The psoric person is also easily fatigued or depressed, always worse in the morning and better when lying down and when scratching the affected areas.

Psoric people share other characteristics. They are often:

- intelligent

- sensitive in mind and body

- philosophical and inventive but unstable, never finishing anything.

- nervous, anxious and often depressed

- hard-working but quickly tiring

- needing to lie down and feeling better for doing so

- always hungry — even after eating

- craving sweet things and unhealthy foods

- suffering from headaches that come on early in the morning and are worse for lying down

- restless, unable to keep still

- feeling better after rest, quiet and sleep

- suffering from skin eruptions

- suffering from bronchial problems and worrying about them

• averse to washing and bathing; wearing dirty clothes

The syphilitic miasm

Syphilis is an insidious disease that reveals itself on the exterior of the body with a characteristic lesion called a *chancre*. The suppression of this prevents the body from dealing with the disease, which ultimately attacks the circulation and nervous system. The syphilitic miasm affects the body structure much more than the psora and often results in bone disease.

This miasm spells destruction. Not only is tissue destroyed, but the person him/herself has a great impulse to destroy. 'Destroy or be destroyed' seems to be the motto of the syphilitic.

The characteristics of the syphilitic miasm are:

• headaches that are worse at night

• nature that is dull, suspicious and cruel

• cold-bloodedness and ruthlessness

• forgetfulness and slow comprehension

• a nature that is melancholic with fixed ideas

• often unreasonable

• ulceration

• sweaty and greasy skin, often with offensive odour

• crusty, oozing eruptions

• bloody discharges

• hair that tends to fall out

• moist scalp

• chilblains and gangrene

• deformed dental arch; irregular and decayed teeth

The sycotic miasm

This is the miasm of gonorrhoea, created when this disease is treated by suppressants. The main feature is greed in all spheres of life, which poisons the person's own existence.

The desire to possess more induces the sycotic to become extremely jealous, vengeful and suspicious, and there is frequent brooding over things. Physically, the miasm generally affects the soft tissues of the body and not the bones, unlike syphilis, which affects both.

The characteristics of the sycotic miasm are:

- vindictiveness, vengefulness and jealousy
- irritability, deceitfulness and cruelty
- violent loss of temper
- poor memory that is especially weak when it comes to remembering names and dates
- disease of the heart valves
- warts and moles
- peptic ulcers and chronic colitis
- aversion to meat
- symptoms that are worse in cold, damp weather
- great sensitivity to changes in the weather
- catarrh in any part of the body
- loss of function in any part of the body — e.g. diabetes
- anaemia
- rheumatism and arthritis
- craving for beer

The tubercular miasm

This results from a combination of the psora and the syphilitic miasm, although some modern homeopaths regard the tubercular miasm as distinct, existing in its own right.

The characteristics of this miasm are:

- continual fatigue

- improvement on lying down
- tendency to get tuberculosis
- weak tendons in ankles and wrists
- corns and callous
- continual hunger
- symptoms worse at high altitude
- greenish-yellow, pus-like sputum, usually with a sweet or salty taste
- tendency towards suicide and mental degeneracy
- tendency towards criminality and insanity
- warts
- catarrhal discharge
- vaginal discharge

HERING'S LAW OF CURE

Homeopaths have found that, in the course of true healing, symptoms and any suppressed manifestations of a miasm will always reappear in the reverse order of their original development. Constantine Hering, the 19th-century American master of homeopathy, encapsulated this principle in his 'Law of Cure'. This states that disease will leave the body:

- from the top downwards
- from the mind to the body
- from inside outwards
- from the main organs to those of lesser importance

HAHNEMANN'S LATER CAREER

Despite (or, perhaps, because of) his genius, Hahnemann was very vain, pompous, irritating and provoking, and therefore an easy target for criticism. His new system of medicine had spread far and wide, with practitioners in other countries reporting good results, and Hahnemann's fame spread, too. As a result, the orthodox medical profession became jealous and wanted to see his reputation destroyed.

The Guild of Apothecaries was well favoured at the time and, so the story goes, they devised a plot to ruin him. A well-known Austrian field marshal, Prince Schwarzenberg, came to Leipzig for professional treatment of what was believed to be an organic infection of the brain (possibly tertiary syphilis). He had been treated by allopathic doctors for some time, but without success. Then the orthodox medics arranged for Prince Schwarzenberg to be placed under Hahnemann's care, but the latter was told nothing about his patient's condition, nor about the previous treatment. He began to treat Schwarzenberg homeopathically, and at first the Prince began to show signs of improvement; then he collapsed suddenly and died.

The orthodox medical practitioners, along with the Guild of Apothecaries, rose in condemnation of Hahnemann and his new methods of treatment, accusing him of negligence and causing the Prince's death. As a result, Hahnemann was prohibited from practising, and unable to prepare and prescribe his remedies. With a large family to support, he was forced to return to translating manuscripts.

When his wife died in 1830, after a brief illness, Hahnemann was grief- stricken. During this time, however, homeopathy was gaining recognition throughout Europe and North America, even though Hahnemann himself was unable to practise.

In 1835, a vivacious Parisienne by the name of Melanie d'Hervilly heard about the famous Hahnemann and came

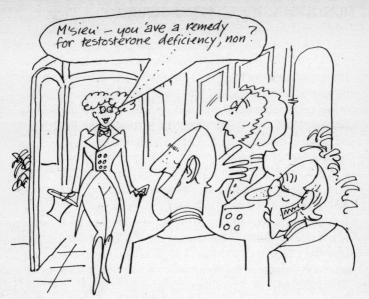

MLLE. MELANIE D'HERVILLY DISGUISED HERSELF AS A BOY IN ORDER TO ENTER THE COMPANY OF THE FAMOUS HAHNEMANN...

up with a plan to meet him: she took the unusual step of disguising herself as a boy in order to enter his company. Her charming youth and beauty captured the heart of the 80-year-old Hahnemann, and the couple were soon married and moved to Paris.

The young Madame Hahnemann had many friends and contacts in high places, including a certain Monsieur Guizot, an influential official from whom she obtained the authority for Hahnemann to practise homeopathy in France. Hahnemann's lifestyle soon changed, and he began to frequent operas and nightclubs. He even made house calls, something he had never done in his early years of practice. In this way, he enjoyed 10 happy and successful years, probably the best of his life, with rich and poor alike flocking to his door. He died in Paris on 2 July 1843 and was buried in the cemetery at Montmartre. However, Hahnemann's fame and popularity continued after his death, and in 1898, he was reburied in Père Lachaise cemetery among the immortals of France.

2.
YOUR FIRST VISIT TO A HOMEOPATH

Your first visit to a homeopath may be prompted by any number of different symptoms. However, the majority of people who seek homeopathic treatment do so because of persistent symptoms that have not responded to conventional allopathic methods. The success rate of homeopathic treatment is very high, and many practitioners excel in chronic cases and those which have not responded to orthodox medicine.

BEFORE THE VISIT

It will be helpful if you note the names of any drugs that you are taking or have taken in the past. If your case is a complicated one, write down the relevant features. The homeopath will be particularly interested in this information, as it will allow him or her to gain a deeper understanding of your case.

Note any unusual symptoms and, if applicable, the times of day when symptoms seem better and/or worse. Note also the *modalities* — that is, anything that improves or worsens your symptoms — and what you do to make yourself more comfortable.

The homeopath will also want to find out more about you as a person — what makes you 'tick'. This kind of information will help the practitioner find the right remedy for your problem, so give the matter some thought before your visit.

THE CONSULTATION

The homeopath's surgery will be much like that of any other health practitioner — a desk and chair for the homeopath, another chair for the patient and an examination couch. There may be shelves containing homeopathic remedies, although most practitioners keep these in a separate room. You will also probably notice the absence of the usual antiseptic odour and clinical appearance of many a conventional surgery. The homeopath's surgery will probably be more homely and have a comfortable atmosphere.

From the moment you enter, the homeopath will be looking for any signs that will indicate the appropriate remedy for you. For example, your handshake may indicate whether you are a confident or an anxious person. After a few preliminary questions to put you at ease, the homeopath will then ask you what brings you to the surgery.

In your own words, describe yourself and your symptoms. Be as complete as possible: it is preferable to tell too much rather than too little about yourself. You will find that the homeopath will be interested in a number of aspects of your problem which your family doctor may have ignored. For instance, you should try to remember and describe the exact nature of any pain that you have experienced:

burning	spreading
bearing down	dull
bursting	throbbing
cramp-like	cutting
boring	deep
shooting	superficial

darting	constant
squeezing	intermittent
splinter-like	moving around
paralyzing	stationary

After you have told why you have come, the process of case-taking begins. This is the real investigation into your complaint. The homeopath will ask a series of searching questions to find out exactly what you are experiencing, why, and what *you* think is the true cause of your malady.

The following are some of the questions you may be asked:

- How do you react to noise?

- Do you dislike being left alone?

- How do you feel when you listen to music?

- Are you frightened of the dark?

- Are you frightened of dogs or any other animals?

- Do thunderstorms affect you?

- Are you often thirsty? If so, do you prefer hot or cold drinks? Do you sip or gulp them?

- Are you always hungry?

- How are you affected by movement and rest?

- Do you dislike hot, cold or damp weather?

- Do you crave meat or any other foods?

- Do you crave hot, spicy food?

- Do you dislike raw food?

- Does the weather affect your symptoms?

- At what times of day do you feel better or worse?

- Are you irritable, anxious or depressed?

- Do you dislike bathing?

- Are you sensitive to criticism?

- Do you cry easily?

Discovering these *modalities* — the things that affect your moods and manner — is very important if the homeopath is to find the right remedy for you. (In cases of first aid, however, the rules don't apply, and the remedy is chosen on a purely symptomatic basis, without regard to the person's mental or physical make-up [see Chapter 4].)

The homeopath will probably also examine you in much the same way as a conventional doctor would. Your pulse and blood pressure will be measured, various parts of your body will be palpated and your heart and breathing will be listened to.

All these questions and examinations can take quite a long time. In fact, most homeopaths allow an hour or more for the first visit and at least half an hour for subsequent ones.

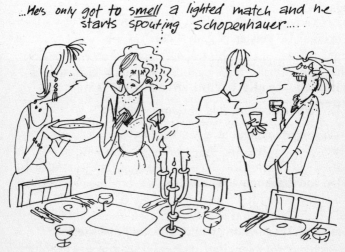

...He's only got to smell a lighted match and he starts spouting Schopenhauer......

'SULPHUR TYPES' CAN BE SUMMED UP AS 'RAGGED PHILOSOPHERS'...

Patient types

Using the information he or she has gathered from talking to you, the homeopath will categorize you according to the remedy that suits your characteristics best. Of course, very few people fit precisely one single remedy and so may share characteristics of other subordinate ones. However, there are those who naturally fit the 'symptom picture' of a particular 'proven' remedy, and these are known as being of a 'constitutional type'; when they are ill, it is their constitutional remedy that will bring the best results.

Examples of four basic 'patient types' are:

● *Sulphur types*
These can be summed up as 'ragged philosophers'. They are untidy, dirty-looking and do not like bathing. They prefer old clothes to new ones, and care nothing for the riches of the world; they have quick tempers. They are also frequently hungry, and experience a sinking feeling in the stomach about 11.00 am. In many respects, the sulphur type is a manifestation of the psora miasm (see pages 19-21), and consequently the remedy sulphur is regarded as the 'Queen of Psora'.

● *Arsenicum types*
Quite different to sulphur types, these are extremely tidy (they cannot bear to see a picture frame tilted by even a millimetre), precise, well-dressed, fastidious and extremely restless.

● *Nux vomica types*
These are irritable and easily aroused, and tend to be workaholics and drink too much alcohol. They are also filled with zest, zeal and vigour — the business tycoons of our time. They often suffer from the effects of over-indulgence, and are easily roused as a result. Their temperatures constantly fluctuate, just like their emotions; even when they have a fever, they are usually chilly.

- *Lycopodium types*

These people are intellectually strong but physically weak. The name refers to the lycopodium plant. In the distant past this was a giant of a tree, but in the process of evolution, it found it hard to adapt to the demands of its changed environment; in order to survive, it gradually shrank in size and, today, it is a mere moss.

Lycopodium types are those who have seen better days, having gradually lost their glory, power and control over life's demands. Consequently, they are cautious and suspicious and lack confidence. Their digestive systems are weak, and although they are often extremely hungry, they feel full very easily. A comparison can be made between the appetites and the sexual natures of lycopodium people: they tend to eat little and often, and seek sexual gratification without responsibilities. They are constantly trying to make up for their inadequacies. They can usually be found in occupations where they have some power or responsibility — for example, politicians, lawyers, clergymen, teachers, civil servants.

Other remedies produce different 'symptom pictures'. For instance, the following demonstrate the ways in which a variety of remedies fit the characteristics found in children:

- *Aurum*

These children lack initiative and 'get up and go', and are often terrified of pain and sensitive to disappointment. Aurum children often sob in their sleep. In boys, one or both testicles are often undescended.

- *Calcarea carbonicum*

These children are fat, fair and flabby, and hot and sweaty on exertion. They have large heads, and are poor at games. They lack initiative and do not venture from where they are told to stay.

- *Capsicum*

These are fat, red-cheeked, red-eared, clumsy children who are slow learners. They have poor memories and are usually labelled as lazy. They suffer from homesickness.

● *Causticum*
These are clumsy children with sallow complexions. They tend to be bedwetters and are liable to warts. However, they are also very sympathetic, and are always upset to see other children crying or otherwise distressed. They tend to get better in damp weather.

● *Chamomilla*
Over-sensitive and very aggressive, these children react to pain with marked resentment and rage. Often one cheek is flushed. Young chamomilla children like to be picked up.

● *China (chinchona, quinine)*
These dislike being handled (the opposite of chamomilla children), and both cheeks may be flushed. They are obstinate and humourless. They tend to pick their noses, and after they vomit, they demand food.

● *Magnesia carbonicum*
The typical Oliver Twist — the great unloved! These children often come from broken homes or have parents who are unhappy together. They are anxious, silent and insecure, and tend to have soft, flabby muscles. They are always nibbling.

● *Medorrhinum*
These children have subnormal intelligence, perhaps as a result of Down's syndrome. They are prone to rheumatism and arthritis and sensitive to reprimands.

● *Phosphorus*
Very intelligent with keen imaginations, these children tend to shrink away from doctors and nurses when taken to hospital. They are afraid of the dark and of thunderstorms, and become anxious if left alone. They are affectionate and responsive.

● *Pulsatilla*
While also afraid of the dark and of being alone, these children — mainly girls — are not as responsive as

phosphorus individuals, but they are warm and loving. Very mild, gentle and yielding, they also cry easily. They like to have a fuss made of them when they are unwell, and are better in the open air; indoors, they like to have a window open. One interesting characteristic is that they like to lie down with their arms stretched above their heads.

● *Sepia*
These children (again, mostly girls) have sallow, greasy skins that tend to sweat profusely. Sepia children are bad mixers and often sulk; they may also wet their beds. They cry easily.

● *Tarantula*
These children are prone to sudden outbursts of destructiveness, especially when not being watched. They are hyperactive, but react badly when given barbiturates as treatment.

● *Thuja occidentalis*
These children have under-average intelligence and are small for their age. Their teeth are crooked, and they may have downy hair on their backs; they are also prone to crops of warts. They are sensitive to music and easily upset. They suffer ill-effects from vaccination.

Although these are only a few of the over 2,000 remedies available to homeopaths, the very wide spectrum of human characteristics can be seen. Unfortunately, the clear-cut cases that have been described do not usually exist in real life. Instead, the homeopath often has only a few slender clues on which to base his or her conclusions.

It is the job of the homeopath to discover a patient's correct 'symptom picture', or *similimum*, and this may take several visits to the surgery. Once yours has been identified, the homeopath will know which remedy will be the most helpful to you. Remember: in homeopathy, the patient is treated, not the disease.

Constitutional types

There is one other consideration that homeopaths must take into account before prescribing a remedy — that is, which type of constitution the patient has. There are two basic ones: the *dynamic* and the *adynamic*.

The body of a person with a *dynamic* constitution has a natural defence system that readily produces antibodies whenever it needs to defend itself against a microscopic intruder. The system learns from experience and remembers how to bring its defences into play whenever necessary.

On the other hand, the body of a person with an *adynamic* constitution reacts slowly to intruders and to change. Its defence system does not protect it effectively, and it does not learn from past experience. As a result, the person is continually susceptible to infection and adversely affected by every change.

People with dynamic constitutions heal easily after operations or injuries. Even when they accidentally become infected by, say, stepping on a poisonous sea urchin or a rusty nail, their bodies immediately react, and healing is automatic. Those with adynamic constitutions, however, can have injections with clean, sterilized needles, with all proper precautions taken, and yet still suffer infections. Their bodies simply do not have enough natural resistance to cope.

SELECTING THE RIGHT REMEDY

This is the homeopath's most difficult task. How efficiently it is done basically depends on his or her knowledge of the *Materia Medica*, the immense book that lists all remedies and all symptoms, with an elaborate system of cross-referencing. For every symptom suffered, there are many remedies, but through a process of elimination, the homeopath will find the one remedy that covers all the symptoms, and this will be the one prescribed.

There are many ways of selecting a remedy. The homeopath may arrive at the correct one by writing down all the patient's various symptoms together with all the possible remedies. Of particular interest will be any strange or peculiar symptoms that a patient may experience. Take, for example, someone with a fever who has a dry mouth but is not thirsty, or feels dizzy when lying down, or likes cold drinks but tends to vomit when they get warm. These are known as *key note* symptoms, and each points to a different remedy. However, the homeopath will not depend solely on these factors. The 'symptom picture' will be seen as a whole, so that physical and mental symptoms are considered along with their modalities (see pages 27 and 30).

A recent method of selecting remedies employs one of the several modern instruments used in bioenergetic medicine (see page 91). These are capable of indicating disturbances within the body by measuring differences in electrical potential on the skin. An alternative method that is a little less objective, but which can be very helpful, is the use of a pendulum, usually made of quartz crystal (see page 90).

Homeopaths who are well versed in the *Materia Medica*, and who have good powers of observation, will often be able to ascertain the necessary remedy within a few seconds of a patient entering the surgery. However, most will still go through the process of case-taking to verify their first impressions.

TAKING THE REMEDY

You may be given a remedy while you are in the surgery. Alternatively, it may be posted or delivered to you — or you may be asked to collect it — together with instructions for use, or you may be given a prescription to be supplied by a homeopathic chemist.

In classic homeopathy, only one remedy is usually prescribed at a time. However, the homeopath might first wish to detoxify your system, in which case you may be given a remedy such as *nux vomica* or *sulphur* (or a combination of these two), to be taken at set intervals. This will clear your system of the influence of drugs, alcohol and other chemical stimulants and depressants before the indicated remedy is prescribed. In addition, some homeopaths will also prescribe biochemical tissue salts, which will aid the working of the remedy (see Scheussler salts, pages 77-83).

Now, let me divulge a little secret! Homeopaths will often tell their patients that they are prescribing two remedies; however, while one consists of the appropriate remedy for the individual, the other will only consist of plain tablets of milk sugar ('sac lac' as they are termed) — in other words a *placebo*. This is done because, very often, only one or two doses of a homeopathic remedy are required for a patient's full recovery, and single doses of some remedies can remain active for a long time — one to six months, or even a whole year — depending on the remedy and its potency. However, many people doubt that such small amounts can be effective, and to reassure their patients, homeopaths give placebos that have no physiological effect whatsoever, although they can have a considerable psychological one!

Since most of the tablets actually containing remedies are sugar based, they are not unpleasant to take. Children in particular seem to look forward to this type of medicine. After a remedy has been prescribed, it is usual to wait for a certain period before a second prescription can be considered.

Do's and don'ts

Most homeopathic remedies come in the form of small tablets that contain little or none of the original substance from which they are derived, but only its dynamic energy, so they can easily lose their effectiveness. To avoid this, it is necessary to follow carefully the homeopath's instructions on how to take a remedy. However, there are some general points that should be remembered:

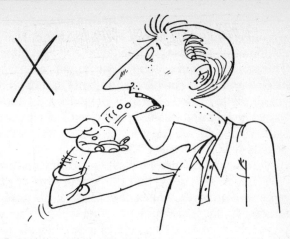

DO NOT HANDLE THE TABLETS ...

- Do not handle the tablets. Pick them up with a clean spoon or drop them into a folded piece of paper or the lid of the bottle and then drop them in your mouth.

- The tablets should be sucked, not swallowed.

- Avoid coffee, peppermint, menthol, eucalyptus and any foods that are highly spiced or strongly seasoned.

- Avoid the use of strong-smelling perfumes, flowers, flavours and so on.

- Do not use toothpaste containing any type of mint (most types are flavoured with peppermint or spearmint). Herbalists and health food shops stock herbal toothpastes, and homeopathic chemists can supply flavourless varieties.

- Avoid eating and drinking for 30 minutes before and after taking a remedy.

Other forms of remedies

Not all homeopathic remedies are taken in tablet form. Some have to be injected; this is more common in Europe,

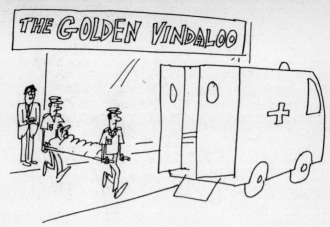

AVOID ANY FOODS THAT ARE HIGHLY SPICED AND STRONGLY
SEASONED ...

although there are a few homeopaths in the UK who use injections. Some remedies also come in liquid form; these may have to be diluted in water and then sipped. Others are prescribed as ointments, to be applied to affected areas.

GENERAL ADVICE

When you visit a homeopath, you will find that, along with the prescribed remedy, you will be given advice on diet and other aspects of healthy living.

. The diet that most homeopaths would recommend is one that is balanced and nutritionally adequate, and which contains plenty of minerals, vitamins and so on. Fruits, vegetables, nuts, seeds, beans, pulses and herbs are the foods that give most nourishment. Meat products, on the other hand, are considered to be 'dead' food, and those who eat them are generally more aggressive and defensive than those who do not.

When taking homeopathic remedies, it is important to

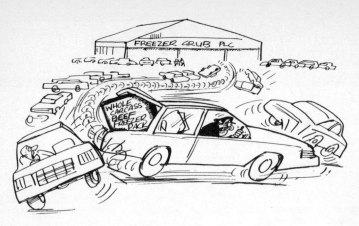

PEOPLE WHO EAT MEAT PRODUCTS ARE GENERALLY
MORE AGGRESSIVE AND DEFENSIVE ...

stick to the diet advised by your homeopath. Certain foods
can affect the action of a remedy, and to deviate from the
practitioner's advice could hinder its effectiveness. Your
homeopath may also suggest that you take certain
nutritional supplements such as vitamins and minerals.

How much food you consume is also important. You
only need to eat enough to supply the body with the energy
and building materials it needs — any more than this and
you will produce an excess of waste materials that will
become toxic and may lead to disease. This is particularly
likely if you become constipated — a healthy person
should have a bowel movement at least once a day. Some
homeopaths will begin treatment by giving their patients
enemas, to clear out the digestive tract; others also
prescribe diuretics (substances that cause the body to lose
fluid), blood purifiers and so on because remedies that are
given afterwards will produce quicker results.

You may also be recommended to fast from time to
time. Homeopaths believe that this helps to cleanse the
body of many impurities and toxins, allowing it to heal.
However, because fasting can be dangerous for some
people, you should only do this under the supervision of a

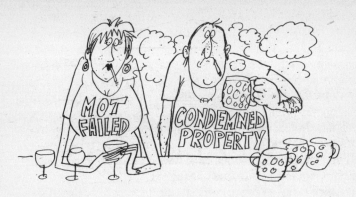

YOUR HOMEOPATH WILL ASK YOU ABOUT ANY UNHEALTHY
HABITS YOU MAY HAVE....

qualified practitioner, who will advise you how to go about
it.

Your homeopath will also ask you about any unhealthy
habits you may have — for example, drinking too much
and smoking. Homeopathic treatment can be enormously
beneficial in helping to alter any negative traits a person
may have inherited, as well as any bad conditioned
reflexes and/or addictions he or she is prone to.

Finally, your own attitude can affect your health *and*
how well your body reacts to any remedies you may be
prescribed. Research has shown that even people with
serious conditions can benefit both physically and
mentally simply by what is known as 'positive thinking'. If
you react negatively towards everything that is done to
help you, and you have a gloomy outlook about your
condition, any treatment that you may undergo will be far
less effective.

AFTER TREATMENT

When you first begin to take a homeopathic remedy, you
may experience a number of strange or unexpected

41

symptoms and sensations. For example, you may have more frequent bowel movements, and the nature of your urine and stools may alter. Your energy level may also change — which will prevent you from living on nervous energy and using up your reserves. Your sleep pattern may be disturbed: you may discover that you sleep more deeply and wake up feeling tired; or you might wake at a certain time of the night or early in the morning. You may develop cravings for foods that you have long forgotten. Symptoms that you once experienced as a child or at some other time in the past may reappear.

Any change in symptoms should be carefully noted so that a new remedy can be selected if necessary. If there are no new symptoms but merely a general improvement, the previous remedy will probably be repeated.

This process can go on for some time, especially in chronic cases where the treatment may be quite protracted — a condition that took many years to develop

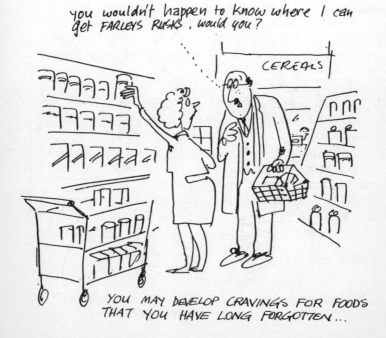

YOU MAY DEVELOP CRAVINGS FOR FOODS THAT YOU HAVE LONG FORGOTTEN...

is unlikely to disappear overnight! Even so, from time to time there are amazing recoveries: the recuperative powers of the body are often quite extraordinary.

Sometimes a low-potency remedy might be prescribed daily for a number of weeks, especially when there is severe damage to organs or other tissues. Remedies of this strength are given particularly to drain major organs such as the liver; this may need to be done before healing can take place.

HOMEOPATHIC AGGRAVATIONS

After starting treatment, a condition may sometimes get worse before getting better. This is called a *homeopathic healing aggravation* — when the potency of a remedy is not correct and it produces symptoms rather than ridding the body of them. You might feel physically ill and a bit anxious; you may even wish you had never gone to a homeopath!

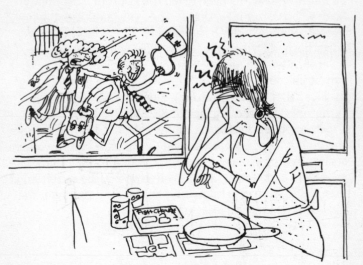

YOUR HOMEOPATH WILL ASK YOU ABOUT THE TIME OF AGGRAVATION...

A skilled homeopath will minimize the chances of an aggravation occurring by choosing the correct potency, but if the one given is not exactly right, the aggravation can be severe. If it becomes unbearable, the homeopath may prescribe another remedy that is quite different from the first, as an antidote. Normally, however, you will simply be prescribed something to slow down the action of the remedy in order to lessen the aggravation.

Symptoms sometimes appear for a short duration at the same time each day or night. Your homeopath will ask you about this *time of aggravation*. If some of your symptoms do behave in this way, it will be possible to prescribe a remedy to help you overcome this, choosing from those known to be effective at particular hours of the day.

A return of old symptoms may occasionally be mistaken for a new condition, but if case-taking has been done carefully, the homeopath will be able to recognize this as a healing process. As a guide, one follows Hering's Law of Cure (see page 23).

A typical example is the man suffering from asthma. As he improves, having been given the appropriate remedy, he develops eczema — that is, the symptoms are moving from inside the body to the outside. Then the rash moves down his body. Any other symptoms will appear in the reverse order to which they were first experienced; so that symptoms suffered in adult life will appear first, followed by those that appeared during adolescence and, finally, symptoms suffered during childhood.

The experience of someone who has been suffering from rheumatic fever is another good example. As improvement occurs, symptoms leave the heart and appear in the shoulders and elbows. As these disappear, the condition is then apparent in the knees and ankles, and finally in the throat, before a complete cure is effected.

FREQUENCY OF TREATMENT

How often you need to see your homeopath will depend very much on the practitioner. Some like to see their patients weekly, others monthly, while still others just tell their patients to book an appointment when they feel they need to.

Clearly, however, there are certain factors that have to be taken into consideration, such as whether the complaint is acute (short-lived) or chronic (long-term). If it is acute, the homeopath might want to see you the next day or in a few hours, depending on the severity of the case. However, if it is a chronic complaint, the intervals between appointments may be considerably longer.

3. QUESTIONS YOU MAY WISH TO ASK

You may have a number of questions you wish to ask before deciding to consult a homeopath professionally. This chapter should help to provide some of the answers.

What can homeopathy offer that orthodox medicine does not?

Many people decide to have homeopathic treatment because they have tried orthodox medicine but have found no relief, or because they are concerned about the amount

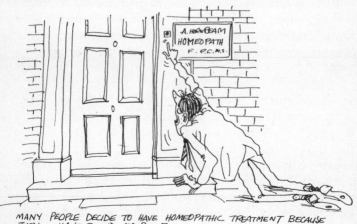

MANY PEOPLE DECIDE TO HAVE HOMEOPATHIC TREATMENT BECAUSE THEY ... HAVE FOUND NO RELIEF

of drugs they are prescribed. Homeopathy tackles the root of a problem; whereas in conventional allopathic treatment, the symptoms are often just suppressed or removed inefficiently, with the underlying cause remaining untouched. Patients who receive homeopathic treatment often report changes in their general outlook as well as in their physical state of health. This shows the importance of treating the mind as well as the body.

However, there are times when orthodox medical treatment is vital — for example, in emergencies such as accidents or where a vital organ is damaged and in a state of crisis. In such cases, homeopathy can still be very helpful used in conjunction with conventional hospital treatment.

Do I really need homeopathy?

It can truthfully be said that we could all benefit from homeopathic treatment because none of us is in perfect health at all times. Homeopathy helps us to be in harmony with nature, which is the basis of good health. If you could carefully select your parents and avoid any hereditary problems, make sure natural childbirth techniques are used when you are born, be nourished with organically grown foods throughout your life, avoid all environmental pollutants and stress, choose the perfect marital partner, remain protected from all harmful social influences and never meet with an accident, you *might* never need homeopathic treatment — or for that matter, any other type!

Is homeopathic treatment safe?

It can happen that a particular individual does not respond to homeopathic treatment, but even so, homeopathy will certainly do no harm. In itself, homeopathy is perfectly safe, although continuing to take a remedy for longer than the prescribed period may lead to a temporary 'proving' (development of symptoms) of that particular remedy. However, the symptoms will disappear as soon as the remedy is stopped.

Will it work?

If homeopathy does not work, then the thousands of eminent physicians who practise this form of medicine are deluding themselves. However, since the majority first enter the field of homeopathy with a critical attitude, it is hardly likely that they are being duped. Although it is true that many people get better without any treatment at all, the consistency with which patients make dramatic recoveries from all kinds of conditions when treated with homeopathy shows how effective it is. Occasionally, there is an aggravation of symptoms in the early stages of treatment (see pages 43-4), but to homeopaths, this is simply another indication that this therapy works! Moreover, it is interesting to note that animals and children, who have no preconceived ideas about homeopathy — all they want is to get better — are some of the best examples of how well homeopathic treatment works.

It is, of course, important to consult a properly qualified homeopath (see below) so that any serious underlying condition will not remain unnoticed. There are people ostensibly practising homeopathy who prescribe remedies that offer relief without actually removing the root cause of a disease. Prescribing in this fashion may never bring about a true homeopathic cure, and can lead to the patient constantly seeking treatment for the same condition and eventually becoming disillusioned with homeopathy.

Are there any conditions which a homeopath cannot treat?

Homeopathy acts best when applied to conditions that are reversible — that is, anything that nature can cure or remove. Homeopathy does not treat disease, as this is only an imbalance of the vital force — when harmony in the vital force is restored, symptoms disappear.

Homeopathy cannot be used in place of surgery, but homeopathic remedies taken in conjunction with surgery can be instrumental in making the latter safer and in hastening post-operative healing. The use of the remedies *arnica* and *hypericum* post-operatively, for example, will help prevent infection. However, it is not uncommon for the maladies of patients being treated homeopathically to disappear and thus make surgery unnecessary.

Since homeopathy is directed at the treatment of a person rather than a disease, it is more relevant to ask whether there are any *people* whom homeopaths cannot treat.

For the most part, the answer is 'no', but it should be remembered that all health practitioners have their failures, particularly when patients refuse to help themselves, continue to have unhealthy lifestyles and do not take prescribed remedies as instructed.

In addition, there are certainly patients who are incurable, but even for these, the quality of their lives can be improved and they can be made comfortable. Because homeopathic remedies also deal with mental symptoms, they can be used to help people with terminal conditions to come to terms with their situation, and more importantly, when death is inevitable homeopathic treatment can help to make it a serene and peaceful experience.

Should I tell my doctor?

This question assumes that your doctor is not a homeopath. In addition to the many homeopaths who are also qualified doctors, a growing number of purely allopathic doctors refer some of their patients to professional homeopaths. However, there are still many GPs who are not sympathetic towards homeopathy. If your doctor is one of these, then you might expose yourself to ridicule by trying to discuss the possibility of homeopathic treatment with him or her. In the end, *you* are responsible for your own health, and it is up to you to decide which kind of medical treatment you wish to receive.

If you decide on homeopathic treatment and your homeopath is not a registered medical practitioner, you should still remain a patient of a medical doctor. As a matter of courtesy, it is a good idea to inform your GP that you are having homeopathic treatment. If this is approached diplomatically, there should be no problem, but if your doctor says it is not a good idea, you have to choose between accepting his advice, ignoring it, or changing your doctor to one more open to the possibilities of homeopathy.

What if I am on medical drugs?

Your homeopath will advise on whether to continue with conventional drug treatment or phase it out. Sometimes homeopathic treatment and other forms of natural medicine stimulate the body's normal functions to the extent that drugs are no longer required in such large doses. More often, homeopathic treatment makes the use of allopathic drugs unnecessary.

As an added bonus, a patient being treated homeopathically for a particular problem will find that his or her whole body benefits. It is not uncommon to experience improvement in all sorts of unexpected areas!

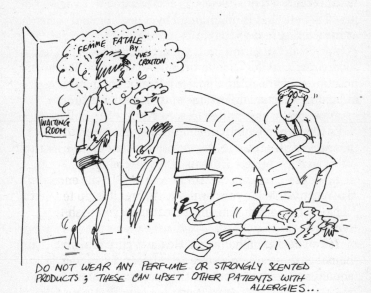

DO NOT WEAR ANY PERFUME OR STRONGLY SCENTED PRODUCTS; THESE CAN UPSET OTHER PATIENTS WITH ALLERGIES...

This is one of the major ways in which homeopathy differs from allopathy.

In the latter, for example, three separate conditions may be treated by three different types of medical drugs, while in homeopathy, one remedy may be all that is needed to restore complete health.

Is there anything I need to do before my visit to a homeopath?

Do not wear any perfume or strongly scented products; these may interfere with the working of any remedy you may be prescribed, and they can upset other patients with allergies. You should also arrange your schedule so that you will not have to rush back to work or home after treatment.

How do I find a qualified practitioner?

It is important to select a properly qualified homeopath — that is, one who practises according to the principles laid down by the founder of homeopathy, Samuel Hahnemann, holds recognized qualifications and is listed in a register of practitioners that is maintained by a professional society or association and available on request to the general public. Such organizations compel their members to be covered by a professional indemnity insurance. These practitioners are entitled to use letters after their names, indicating their qualifications and their registration with an appropriate association or society.

To find a homeopath in your locality, contact one of these organizations (see pages 95-6 for Useful Addresses), your Citizens' Advice Bureau or your local library.

How much will treatment cost?

Not all homeopaths charge the same fees; for example, those who practise in cities and large towns tend to charge more because of higher rents. However, if you are a private patient, the fee will probably be between £20 and £30 (sometimes a little more) for the first visit, which can last much more than an hour. If you cannot afford this, you may be able to find a registered medical practitioner practising homeopathy within the National Health Service, although there are relatively few of these. In addition, there are a few homeopathic hospitals where treatment is free, and which you can attend as an out-patient. (See page 000 for Useful Addresses.)

Do I need a referral to attend a homeopathic hospital?

As a rule, hospitals like to have letters from patients' GPs before they attend. However, if it is impossible to obtain one — perhaps because your family doctor is opposed to homeopathic medicine — you can explain the problem to the relevant person at the hospital.

Can fees be recovered from medical insurance?

Very often this is possible, particularly if the homeopath is also a medically qualified doctor. There are now also insurance schemes specifically designed to cover treatment provided by what are commonly known as 'complementary medical practitioners', which include homeopaths. Check your own insurance cover, and talk to your insurance broker if you are interested in one of the 'complementary medicine' schemes.

Will the homeopath visit me at home?

Most homeopaths make house calls in emergencies only. However, a few do carry out regular home visits.

Will the homeopath explain what is wrong with me?

A properly qualified homeopath will certainly be able to tell you what is wrong with you in terms of normal anatomy and physiology. However, your physical symptoms are only pointers to the right remedy. Your whole being — your physical and mental make-up and your modalities (see pages 27 and 30) — will be considered in order to find the remedy that will aid the cure. This is why you may be referred to by the name of that remedy — for example, as a 'pulsatilla' — rather than as someone suffering from, say, arthritis or laryngitis.

What is the difference between homeopathy and herbalism?

There are many differences between these two therapies. In the first place, although many homeopathic remedies are herbal in origin, others are derived from minerals and even animals. Examples of the latter are *lachesis* (snake venom), *apis* (bee), *formica* (ant), *sepia* (cuttlefish) and *tarantula* (spider). Moreover, some of the remedies, known as *nosodes*, are made up of diseased tissue.

The most important difference is that homeopathic treatment is based on the Law of Similars (treating like with like); herbalism is not. Lastly, herbalists always use physiological or material doses of the herbs, whereas homeopaths use remedies which are potentized drugs (see pages 15-17). However, there is a form of homeopathy — *complex homeopathy* — that involves mixtures of remedies in low potency. In this respect, it is similar to herbal medicine.

What are Scheussler salts?

These are the 12 biochemical tissue salts that have been found to remain as ash when the body is cremated. The 19th-century German doctor, Wilhelm Scheussler, who established this system of medicine, believed that these salts must form an essential component of a healthy diet, and that the reason why diseases arose was due to deficiencies of these salts. By taking them in homeopathic potencies, the body is encouraged to absorb them better. (For more information, see pages 77-83).

4.
HOMEOPATHIC FIRST AID

Under normal circumstances, a homeopathic remedy that matches the individual's physical and mental characteristics is chosen; symptoms of any illness are generally only a small part of the total picture. However, when treating accidental injuries such as cuts and sprains or providing temporary relief from the pain of headaches, arthritis and cystitis, remedies are chosen on the basis of the symptoms alone.

FIRST AID REMEDIES

The following are the remedies primarily used in homeopathic first aid. These are available (individually or in first aid kits) from homeopathic chemists and some health food shops.

Each entry below gives: the symptoms that the remedy will alleviate; an indication, where appropriate, of the substance (plant, animal, mineral) from which the remedy is derived; and information as to which things will make the symptoms better or worse, so that the right remedy can be chosen. How these remedies can be used to treat individual conditions is discussed on pages 67-75.

Aconitum (aconite)
Indicated for: physical and mental restlessness; fear, violent emotional shock; first stage of congestion; inflammation.

Better: in open air.
Worse: in warm rooms; in evening and at night; when
lying on affected part; in cold, dry wind.

Apis mellifica (honey bee)

Indicated for: insect and animal bites and puncture
wounds; oedema (swelling due to accumulation of fluid in
the tissues); jealousy, fright, anger, grief; burning pains;
difficult urination, which is hot and burning.
Better: from bathing; in open air.
Worse: in late afternoon; from heat; when touched; after
sleep. Symptoms aggravated between 4.00 and 6.00 pm.

Arnica montana

Indicated for: bruises, muscle sprains, falls, fractures, etc.
Advisable to take after dental or surgical operations to
prevent infection and relieve pain.
Better: when lying down.
Worse: when touched; in motion; in damp cold.

Argentum metallicum (silver)

Indicated for: loss of voice, especially in singers; sore
throat with jelly-like mucus, cough, leucorrhoea (vaginal
discharge).
Better: in open air; when lying down.
Worse: when riding in a vehicle; talking; singing; being
touched or pressed.

Argentum nitricum (silver nitrate)

Indicated for: disease due to long mental exertion;
withered skin and premature ageing; eyelids sore and
gummy in the morning; flatulence and indigestion with
belching at meals; diarrhoea with green mucus which
looks like chopped spinach; impotence (erection fails when
coitus is attempted).
Better: when cold; in fresh air; with pressure.
Worse: after cold food at night; with unusual mental
exertion; when warm; after eating sweets; on left side.

Arsenicum album (arsenic)

Indicated for: restlessness, anxiety and fear; prostration; gastro-enteritis and food poisoning; burning pains; aversion to sight and smell of food.

Better: in cool air; when kept warm; when heat is applied to affected parts.

Worse: in cold and wet weather; at midnight. Symptoms aggravated between 1.00 and 2.00 am.

Belladonna (deadly nightshade)

Indicated for: severe, sharp, throbbing, pulsating, shooting pains; painful spasms with jerking and convulsions; fevers with inflammation of the joints; bursting headaches; vertigo; catarrhal fever.

Better: when semi-erect.

Worse: in draughts; in the afternoon; when lying down and touched; in a noisy environment. Symptoms aggravated between 3.00 and 10.00 pm and at midnight.

Bryonia (bryony)

Indicated for: rheumatism and lower back pain; irritability; chestiness; dry, painful, violent cough; bronchitis; fevers; gastric problems; constipation.

Better: when lying on painful side; when resting; on pressure.

Worse: on the least motion; when eating in the morning. Symptoms aggravated at 3.00 am and 9.00 pm.

Cantharis (Spanish fly)

Indicated for: all burns and scalds; urinary tract conditions; sunburn; gnat bites, styes in the eye.

Better: when rubbed.

Worse: when cold water or hot coffee is drunk; when touched; on urination.

Calendula officinalis (marigold)

Indicated for: wounds and cuts, to promote healing and prevent suppuration; deafness; catarrhal conditions.

Worse: in damp, heavy cloudy weather.

Camphor

Indicated for: gastro-enteritis; sudden unconsciousness; convulsions; fainting.
Better: in warm air; when drinking cold water.
Worse: when in motion; at night; in cold air.

Carbo-veg

Indicated for: indigestion with flatulence ('wind'); poor digestion; acidity and heartburn; low blood pressure; bad circulation, especially when skin turns blue with cold; breathlessness; extreme weakness; spongy, ulcerated gums.
Better: when fanned, cold and/or wind is brought up.
Worse: after eating rich food; in warm, damp weather; after drinking milk, wine and coffee; during the evening and night. Symptoms aggravated between 4.00 and 5.00 pm and before midnight.

Causticum

Indicated for: stiffness; tearing, drawing and shooting pains; painful cracking of the knee when walking; dry, hollow cough; sore throat; hoarseness; frequent desire to urinate; uncontrolled urination in children and elderly.
Better: in damp wet weather; in warm bed.
Worse: in dry, cold winds; from motion.

Chamomilla (German chamomile)

Indicated for: fretful children who are quiet only when picked up; peevish, restless and colicky children; people who are irritable, sensitive, hot, thirsty and numb; when one cheek is red.
Better: in damp weather; in warm bed.
Worse: in dry, cold winds; when in motion.

China (chinchona bark, quinine)

Indicated for: intermittent fevers; all symptoms brought on by loss of vital fluids — for example, during haemorrhages, diarrhoea, vomiting.
Better: in heat; on pressure; in open air.
Worse: in draughts; at night.

Crocus sativa (saffron)

Indicated for: frequent and extreme emotional changes; nosebleeds with black, stringy, sticky blood.
Better: in the open air.
Worse: on lying down; in hot weather; in a warm room; in the morning; with fasting; before breakfast; when looking fixedly at an object.

Crotalus horridus (rattlesnake venom)

Indicated for: bleeding, especially from eyes, nose, mouth and every other orifice in the body; severe jaundice; severe prostration; right-side paralysis.
Worse: on the right side; in the open air; in evening and morning; in spring; at the onset of warm weather; on waking; in damp and wet weather; on jarring.

Drosera rotundifolia (sundew)

Indicated for: whooping cough with violent paroxysms following one another rapidly; clergyman's sore throat with rough, scraping dry sensation; bed feels too hard.
Better: from pressure with the hands.
Worse: after midnight; when lying down; on getting warm in bed; on drinking; on singing; on laughing.

Echinacea (purple cornflower)

Indicated for: septic conditions; tiredness; meningitis; recurrent boils.

Gelsemium sempervirens (yellow jasmine)

Indicated for: paralysis; prostration with dizziness; drowsiness and trembling; muscular weakness; nervous, hysterical disposition.
Better: on bending forward; with profuse urination; in open air; when taking stimulants; with continued motion.
Worse: in damp weather; in fog; before a thunderstorm; with emotion or excitement; on receiving bad news; when smoking tobacco; at about 10.00 am.

Graphites (black lead)

Indicated for: fat, chilly and constipated people; suited to women who are inclined to obesity and chronic constipation; nausea and vomiting in the morning during periods.
Better: in the dark; from wrapping up.
Worse: for warmth; at night; during and after periods.

Hamamelis (witch hazel)

Indicated for: varicose veins; congestion of and bleeding from veins; bleeding piles; chilblains; for pain after operations; bruised soreness from injuries; tired, painful muscles and joints.
Better: in open air.
Worse: when touched; in heat; in moist air.

Hypericum (St John's wort)

Indicated for: painful cuts and wounds, including puncture wounds; injury to spine, especially to coccyx and nerve ends; horsefly bites; painful corns and bunions. Prevents pain and tetanus.
Better: when bending head backwards.
Worse: in cold and dampness; when touched.

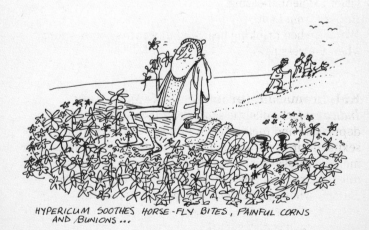

HYPERICUM SOOTHES HORSE-FLY BITES, PAINFUL CORNS AND BUNIONS ...

Ignatia

Indicated for: ill effects of grief, trauma, injury, shock and disappointment; hysteria, changeable moods; weepiness and sadness; twitching; anal problems; dry, spasmodic coughing.

Better: from hard pressure; when lying on painful side; on profuse urination.

Worse: from slightest touch; when drinking coffee; when smoking.

Ipecacuanha (ipecac root)

Indicated for: irritation and spasms in the chest and stomach with haemorrhages; fermented, green and slimy stools; asthma; consistent nausea and vomiting; vomiting during pregnancy; hoarseness; whooping cough.

Worse: from lying down; in moist, warm wind; when eating veal.

Kali bichromicum (bichromate of potash)

Indicated for: paralysis with weakness; cirrhosis of the liver; gastric disturbances (including ulcers); problems of the heart, liver and kidneys; vertigo; nausea; blurred vision; violent sneezing.

Better: from heat.

Worse: when drinking beer; in hot weather; in morning; when undressing.

Kali bromatum (bromide of potash)

Indicated for: epileptic seizures; anaemia; insanity; depression and melancholia; fidgety hands; inappropriate sexual desires; paralysis; intense thirst with vomiting after meals; profuse urination in diabetes; acne; sleeplessness due to worry and grief; grinding of teeth during sleep.

Better: when physically and mentally occupied.

Lachesis (venom of bushmaster snake, or surucucu)

Indicated for: delirium with much trembling and confusion; ill effects of suppressed discharges; left-sided sore throat; offensive stools; constricted anus; intense excitement of sexual organs; dry, suffocating, tickling cough.

Better: from discharges and warm applications.

Worse: after sleep; on left side; on closing eyes; on pressure; after hot drinks.

Ledum palustre (marsh tea)

Indicated for: all animal bites; craving for whisky. Useful as an anti-tetanus remedy, and particularly helpful for wounds caused by pointed instruments.

Better: when feet put in cold water.

Worse: in heat of warm bed; at night.

Lobelia inflata (Indian tobacco)

Indicated for: nausea and vomiting, accompanied by great relaxation of the muscular system and profuse salivation; deafness due to suppressed discharges; burning, acrid taste in mouth; shortness of breath; heartburn.

Better: from rapid motion; in evening; from warmth.

Worse: from cold washing; taking tobacco; in the afternoon; on slightest motion.

Lycopodium (club moss)

Indicated for: sadness; weak memory; loss of self-confidence; flatulence; downward pressure in intestines; extreme hunger although eating a little makes the stomach full; right-sided throat problems; excessive urination; impotence and premature ejaculation; palpitations at night; burning between shoulder blades; inability to lie on left side; offensive perspiration from feet and armpits; abscesses beneath skin, acne and violent itching.

Better: from motion; taking hot food and drink; on being uncovered.

Worse: on right side; between 4.00—8.00 pm; in a warm room.

Medorrhinum (gonorrhoeal virus)

Indicated for: chronic rheumatism, stunted growth; chronic catarrhal conditions; trembling all over the body; swollen, sore and stiff ankles; weak memory.
Better: from lying on stomach; in damp weather; by the sea.
Worse: from sunrise to sunset; on application of heat; when thinking of ailment.

Mercurius (quicksilver)

Indicated for: glandular swellings, ulcers, moist tongue, slimy mucous membranes; spongy, swollen or bleeding gums; offensive breath; profuse sweating; soreness in the bones; burning pains; intense thirst for cold drink; weak memory; bleeding; tremors; abscesses; profuse diarrhoea.
Worse: at night; in damp weather; when lying on right side; on perspiring; in warm bed.
Note: There are many types of mercurius. *Merc. solubilis* and *merc. virus* are very similar, but it is claimed that *merc. vir.* is better adapted to men and *merc. sol.* to women; *merc. sol.* is also a better remedy for skin problems and dribbling due to excess salivation. *Merc. corrosivus* is especially indicated for an unproductive urge to defecate, when urine is passed in drops with intense pains, for inflammation of the throat with burning pains, and for swollen gums that bleed easily.

Nux moschata (nutmeg)

Indicated for: intense drowsiness; visual disturbance (objects look larger); intense dryness of the mouth and mucous membranes; moodiness; confusion; weak memory; oversensitivity to smell; excessively bloated stomach with flatulence; fainting when defecating.
Better: from warmth; in dry weather.
Worse: from cold food; in cold wind; during cold washing; lying on painful side.

Nux vomica (poison-nut)

Indicated for: detoxifying the body; irritability; nervousness; oversensitivity; addiction to stimulants, narcotic drugs and highly spiced food; ill effects of rich, fatty, indigestible foods, wine and other alcoholic drinks; fainting due to strong odours; frequent and ineffectual desire to pass stools; twitching, spasms and chilliness.
Better: in the evening; at rest; in wet weather; under strong pressure.
Worse: under mental exertion; taking stimulants; after eating; when touched; in morning.

Pulsatilla ('weather-cock remedy')

Indicated for: sadness; weepiness, passivity and irritability; soft and flabby muscles; moodiness; pains that rapidly change location; intermittent haemorrhages; stomach easily disturbed by rich, fatty food; light or suppressed periods.
Better: in open air, after cold food and drink; from motion; with cold applications.
Worse: from crying; in heat; after eating rich food; in warm room.

Phosphoricum (phosphorus)

Indicated for: bleeding; physical and mental hyper-sensitivity; dry coughs, hoarseness, loss of voice.
Better: after eating cold food; in open air.
Worse: after ingesting warm food and drink; in the evening.

Rhus tox (icodendron) (poisonsumac)

Indicated for: rheumatic and arthritic aches and pains; chicken pox; herpes; lower back pain; sciatica; shingles; measles; intolerable itching of skin; fear, anxiety, restlessness.
Better: on gentle motion; on application of heat; in warm weather.
Worse: in cold and wet weather; during rest; after midnight.

Ruta graveolens (rue)

Indicated for: bone injuries and fractures; sprains, dislocations; eye injuries (including eyestrain); rheumatism and general aches and pains.
Better: in warm weather; on application of heat; on gentle motion.
Worse: in cold, damp weather; when lying down.

Sabina (savine)

Indicated for: haemorrhages and blood clots in sacrum and pubic area; habitual miscarriage around third month; violent, pulsating pains which emanate from the back, travel between sacrum and pubis or ascend from the vagina; air hunger with a desire to open windows; intolerance to music.
Better: in fresh air.
Worse: from heat and motion.

Sepia (cuttle-fish ink)

Indicated for: all 'women's complaints' (vaginal discharge, prolapsed uterus, painful periods, morning sickness); violent colic pains with fainting sensations.
Better: during exercise and dancing; in heat of warm bed; on pressure; when heat applied; when limbs drawn up.
Worse: at noon and in evening; when washed; when feet become wet.

Spongia tosta (roasted sponge)

Indicated for: anxiety and difficulties in breathing, along with exhaustion and heaviness of the body, made worse by slightest exertion causing blood to rush into chest and face; excessive thirst with hunger and excitement; dry, barking cough; sensation of a plug in the larynx; wakefulness at night with fear and anxiety causing a feeling of suffocation.
Better: from descending wind; when lying with head low.
Worse: from ascending wind; before midnight.

Staphisagria (stavesacre)

Indicated for: toothache; backache; recurring styes;
healing post-operative scars, and any clean cut or incision;
suppressed anger and grief; warts, especially around
genitalia.
Better: in heat; at night.
Worse: due to loss of fluids, anger, grief.

Sulphur

Indicated for: dry, scaly skin with eruptions causing
burning and intolerable itching; thirst; intolerance to milk;
weakness and faintness around 11.00 am; sensitivity to
smell, including own odour.
Better: in dry, warm weather; when lying on right side
and drawing up affected limb.
Worse: from heat, washing, alcohol, stimulants and
standing.

Symphytum (comfrey) *Indicated for:* cases of
fractures and injury to cartilage, to help knitting of bones;
injuries to the eye from blunt objects or from a blow.

Urtica urens (stinging nettle)

Indicated for: rheumatism accompanied by psoric
eruptions; burning, itching skin, generally worse from
cold; ill effects of eating shellfish; gouty symptoms;
chronic diarrhoea with a lot of mucus.
Worse: from cool air; when touched.

Some of the various tissue salts (see pages 77-83) and
the Bach flower remedies (see pages 83-7) may also be
used in first aid. There is also a combination of three
remedies — *aconitum, belladonna* and *chamomilla* —
which is suitable for treating fevers and a majority of
childhood maladies. Known as 'ABC', it can be purchased
from most homeopathic chemists.

CONDITIONS HELPED BY HOMEOPATHIC FIRST AID

Note: When no potency is given for a particular remedy, you should try the 6th or the 30th potency on the centesimal scale (see page 16). Any potency higher than 30c should not be taken unless it has been prescribed by a qualified homeopath.

Sometimes drops of the homeopathic remedy in liquid form — known as the *mother tincture* — are added to water or another substance to make a lotion or ointment.

Arthritis

When joints are inflamed, painful and swollen, and symptoms are relieved by movement, *rhus tox* 30c will be very helpful.

In cases of arthritis where there is constriction of the joints and symptoms are only relieved if the joints remain still, *bryonia* will reduce pain and help to improve the quality of life.

Bruises

The best remedy for all forms of bruising is *arnica montana*, which can be applied as an ointment or lotion. (To prepare a lotion, add five drops of arnica mother tincture to 5 fluid ounces of boiled and cooled water.) However, arnica should not be applied if the skin is broken; tablets of arnica 6c or 30c, taken by mouth, are very effective.

In more serious cases of bruising, apply a cold compress to the affected parts and, at the same time, take arnica 6c or 30c approximately every four hours until healing is complete or the aches and pains have subsided. When there is a bruise accompanying a sprained muscle or tendon, you can alternate between arnica 30c and *ruta grav* 6c on a four-hourly basis until you are satisfied that nature can take over and do the rest.

Burns
Deep burns should be swabbed with oil of turpentine or
hypericum lotion or cream; honey may also be applied.
The burn should then be covered with dry, sterile gauze
which may be moistened with hypericum lotion. *Cantharis*
30c or *urtica urens* 30c may be taken by mouth at frequent
intervals.

Colds
Violent sneezing with a dry cough, and colds brought on
due to exposure to draughts both call for *aconitum.*

Colds caused by sudden changes from heat to cold,
resulting in a throbbing headache, obstruction of the nose
and pain in the throat, suggest *chamomilla.*

Colds involving a sore, runny nose with acrid discharge
indicate *arsenicum album.*

Constipation
This is a condition suffered by most people at some time in
their lives. The laxatives readily available do not always
work and they produce many unnecessary side-effects. A
simple and harmless homeopathic remedy may do the
trick. One tablet of *nux vomica* 30c taken three times a
day for a day or two should be enough to bring about a
bowel motion. However, there are many remedies for this
complaint, and if nux vomica does not work in a short
time, consult your homeopath.

If stools are large and painful, try *sulphur.* If they are
hard to expel because they come out halfway and then
recede, *silicea* (a Scheussler salt, see pages 77-83) may
be the answer.

Coughs
When the cough is dry and painful, is better from pressure
and the patient does not like being moved, *bryonia* may
help.

For violent attacks of coughing, which may or may not
be whooping cough, take *drosera.*

For wheezing coughs that improve when the skin becomes moist, take *spongia*.

For coughing with vomiting, when the body becomes stiff and the face blue, the patient becomes breathless if he or she moves, and symptoms become worse at night, *ipecacuanha* should be taken.

When coughing does not bring up mucus, even though there is a lot of it in the airways, try *kali bichromicum*.

Cuts, wounds and animal bites

For small cuts, the best treatment is *calendula*. After washing the cut under running water or with soap and water, apply a little calendula ointment. Alternatively, you can use calendula lotion, made by adding five drops of calendula mother tincture to 10 fluid ounces (about one cupful) of boiled and cooled water. *Hypercal* (a mixture of calendula and *hypericum*) may be used instead.

For deep cuts and wounds, first remove any visible debris from the surface. The cut should then be swabbed with hypericum or hypercal lotion. After cleansing the wound, apply a sterile gauze dressing. Moisten this with the lotion, keeping it moist until the wound has healed. Take tablets of hypericum 30c twice a day (preferably one in the morning and one at night), or one tablet of hypericum 6x every four hours until healing is complete.

Puncture wounds (such as those made by stepping on a nail) and animal bites can be treated with hypericum lotion or ointment or with a lotion made from *ledum palustre*. Ledum 30c tablets should then be taken, one every four hours for two or three days.

Cystitis

If there is an acute urinary infection, with a sensation of motion in the bladder and continuous passing of urine, take *belladonna*.

When there is an intolerable urge to urinate, the urine feels hot and is passed in drops, with violent cutting and burning pains, try *cantharis*.

When there are burning pains in the urethra which last long after urine is passed, *sulphur* is recommended.

Diarrhoea

Diarrhoea brought on by anticipation, fear, worry and so on may respond to *argentum nitricum*.

When symptoms are caused by fear and worry, and the person has difficulty coping with life's demands, *gelsemium* is often helpful.

For diarrhoea with colic — stools that feel as if they are burning as they are passed, plus abdominal cramps and a cutting pain in rectum — *lycopodium* is recommended.

Sulphur is suggested for early-morning diarrhoea which drives the patient out of bed, and for stools that are fetid or sour smelling or contain undigested foods.

For diarrhoea due to food poisoning, especially that caused by seafood, try *arsenicum album*.

Earache

When the ear is red and hot and the pain is of a throbbing nature, *belladonna* should be taken.

Eczema

When the skin is hard, dry and cracked in the folds, with a lot of burning and itching, *sulphur* 6c taken every four hours, or sulphur 30c taken once a day, will help to relieve the symptoms. As sulphur is an anti-psoric remedy (see page 31), it may even cure the eczema.

Sometimes small blisters (resembling measles) appear on the skin, which burst and then dry up, causing itching and swelling. *Rhus tox* 30c, taken once a day, may be very helpful. Occasionally the condition may worsen when this remedy is taken; if this happens, discontinue the remedy and see how you feel in a day or two. If the skin problem was acute, it may then disappear completely, but if it is chronic, it is wise to try taking the remedy again; if the aggravation reappears, stop taking the rhus tox and ask your homeopath for advice.

When the skin cracks and weeps, *graphites* 6c or 30c

will be most useful. If the eczema is mostly on the hairline, *nat mur* (a Scheussler salt, see pages 80-81) is indicated.

Fear and shock
There are many different kinds of traumatic events that can bring on fear or shock. The following list provides the different remedies suitable to the varying qualities of these:

- Sudden death in the family, or any other shock: *ignatia, aconitum, rescue remedy* (see page 87).

- After an accident, fall or injury: *arnica montana.*

- Terror: *arsenicum album.*

- Fear of exams: *gelsemium.*

- Fear of crowds, accompanied by a feeling that something terrible is going to happen: *ferr phos* (a Scheussler salt, see pages 80-81). *argentum nitricum.*

Fever
When the body is hot and dry and the face is red, and the fever is accompanied by cold 'waves' that pass through the body, and by thirst and restlessness, *aconitum* is recommended.

For a very high fever with burning, pungent heat but no thirst, take *belladonna.*

When a fever makes the person sensitive, irritable, hot, numb and thirsty, the tongue is yellow, and there is a bitter taste in mouth, take *chamomilla.*

Fractures
In the case of fractures, it is useful to give a dose of *arnica* 30c (or 200c, if this is available). *Hypericum* 30c may be given if the skin is bruised. To accelerate healing, *symphytum officinalis* 6x (comfrey) should be taken two or three times a day. *Ruta grav* 30c or 6c may also be taken for tendon damage.

Headache

Belladonna is recommended when there is vertigo with staggering and trembling, a sense of stupor, fullness in the head with violent beating of the carotid arteries, and the patient does not want to be moved.

Nux vomica is the remedy of choice when there is vertigo with dizziness and a feeling of bewilderment, clouded vision and buzzing in the ears, especially if the patient is quick, hasty and addicted to coffee.

Take *pulsatilla* if vertigo is worse after stooping, causing temporary blindness; the patient staggers with a fear of falling; the pains are one sided, pulsating and shooting in nature; the headache feels as if it is coming from the stomach; and there is numbness in the limbs.

Insect bites

Hypercal tincture may be applied direct, or a preparation made with *pyrethrum*. The latter is particularly effective in the case of mosquito and gnat bites.

Nausea

During pregnancy, a variety of types of nausea may be experienced, with a corresponding number of remedies required:

- At the sight and smell of food: *arsenicum album*.

- With fainting and weakness: *lobelia inflata*.

- Very frequent vomiting: *medorrhinum*.

- Empty feeling, nausea in the morning before eating, cravings for vinegar and acidic foods: *sepia*.

Nose bleeds

The first choice of remedy for nose bleeds is *hamamelis*. However, there are a number of alternatives:

- Brought on by coughing: *phosphorus*.

- With absent periods: *lachesis, pulsatilla*.

- On blowing nose: *arg-met.*

- During fever: *rhus-tox.*

- With vertigo: *belladonna, lachesis, sulphur.*

- In young girls: *crocus sativa.*

- In women: *phosphorus.*

Period problems
Again, there are a number of alternatives:

- If there is copious bleeding, take *nux vomica, phosphorus* or *sabina.*

- If periods are irregular, try *belladonna, nux mos, pulsatilla.*

- If periods are absent, *pulsatilla* is recommended.

- For painful periods, try *chamomilla, pulsatilla* or *sulphur.*

- When periods are brought on by emotional upset, take *chamomilla.*

Snake bites
Apply one or two drops of hypericum tincture; take the Bach flower '*rescue remedy*' (see page 87) followed by *ledum* 30c. If the skin turns blue and there is bleeding, take *lachesis* 30c. If there is rapid development of toxic symptoms (including swelling, discoloration and bleeding), take *crotalus horridus* 30c. If there is infection, gangrene or a foul-smelling discharge, take *echinacea* 6x. Where there is a livid colour and parts of the body are cold and numb with violent pains and tremors, or if the casualty is comatose with a dusky face and pallor around the mouth, give *carbonicum, acidum* 30c (placing a few drops of this under the tongue).

Toothache

Toothache that is worse when hot and cold food and drink is consumed, and generally feels better when the cheeks are rubbed, can be relieved by *mercurius solubilus*. However, when the pains are radiating and the teeth are loose, *merc* is a better option.

Silicea (a Scheussler salt, see pages 80-81). Should be taken for toothache resulting from an abscess at the roots.

For toothache caused by severely decayed and crumbling teeth, take *staphisagria*.

Vomiting

Different remedies will suit different situations:

- Vomiting easily: *arsenicum album, chamomilla*.

- After eating or from emotions: *kali bromatum*.

- Retching and vomiting with coughing: *phosphorus*.

- With headache: *ipecacuanha, nux vomica, pulsatilla*.

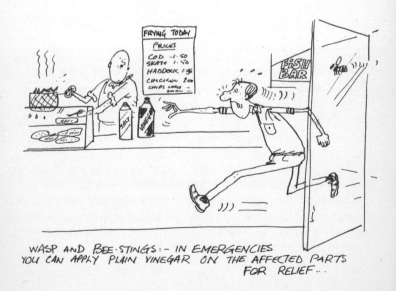

WASP AND BEE·STINGS :- IN EMERGENCIES YOU CAN APPLY PLAIN VINEGAR ON THE AFFECTED PARTS FOR RELIEF...

Wasp and bee stings *Ledum* tincture and *apis* may be applied directly on to the affected area. Ledum 6c or apis 6c may also be taken by mouth with or without the application of any ointment or tincture. In emergencies, you can apply plain vinegar on the affected parts for relief.

5.
HOMEOPATHY AND OTHER THERAPIES

As we have seen, homeopathy cannot be used as a substitute if a surgical operation is necessary. In addition, many homeopaths also recognize other therapies as useful adjuncts to homeopathic treatment. For example, if there is a problem with bones and/or muscles, one of the manipulative therapies — osteopathy and chiropractic — will be recommended; a homeopathic remedy may be given when this treatment is finished, to prevent the problem from recurring. Wise homeopathic practitioners realize their limitations and know when to advise a change of therapy.

In addition, certain forms of complementary medicine are frequently employed alongside homeopathic treatment — notably Scheussler salts, Bach flower remedies and acupuncture. These and other therapies, as well as certain specialized forms of homeopathy itself, are discussed in the following pages.

SCHEUSSLER SALTS (TISSUE SALTS)

Thirty years after Hahnemann's death, when homeopathy had been flourishing for quite a time, an article appeared, entitled 'Abridged Homeopathic Therapeutics' and written by another German doctor, Wilhelm Scheussler. In this paper, Dr Scheussler proposed a system — which he termed 'biochemistry' — in which the 12 inorganic chemical compounds, or 'tissue salts' (mineral salts), that make up the human body were to be used as therapeutic agents. His main thesis was that disease resulted from deficiencies of these substances, either because they were lacking in the diet or, much more commonly, because the body did not absorb them correctly.

This paper was followed by six more, and they all provoked tremendous interest. They also incurred the wrath of classical homeopaths for daring to question the teachings of Hahnemann. Although, in many ways, the latter's great discoveries were enshrined in Scheussler's hypothesis, there was a parting of the ways because of Scheussler's belief that only the 12 tissue salts (which are minerals or mineral compounds) should be used as remedies. In fact, he argued that other remedies employed by homeopaths worked only because of the tissue salts they contained, stating that it is a physiological fact that both the structure and vitality of the organs of the body are dependent upon its inorganic constituents.

He went on to suggest that any deficiency of these substances would result in the body's inability to repair itself. This deficiency could be rectified by administering the required mineral salts in small quantities.

The 12 tissue salts that he identified, often the 'biochemical remedies', are:

Calc fluor (calcium fluoride)
Calc phos (calcium phosphate)
Calc sulph (calcium sulphate)
Ferr phos (iron phosphate)
Kali mur (potassium chloride)
Kali phos (potassium phosphate)
Kali sulph (potassium sulphate)
Mag phos (magnesium phosphate)
Nat mur (sodium chloride)
Nat phos (sodium phosphate)

Nat sulph (sodium sulphate)
Silicea (silica)

Scheussler's theory

Disease is unnatural, and nature provides what is required for good health. This is dependent on the right quantity and distribution of both organic and inorganic constituents of the body.

Should a deficiency of one or more of the tissue salts occur, an abnormal condition would arise. Every disease to which human beings are prone, every symptom, every pain and every unpleasant sensation are all the result of a lack of one or more of these compounds.

All life begins in the soil, and all animal life is dependent upon the plant kingdom. Only plants are able to absorb the nutrients direct from the soil and convert them into organic food for animals and humans. The fundamental law of health is that there must be a healthy soil for healthy vegetation to grow. Nowadays, unfortunately, soil is often polluted by huge quantities of synthetic chemicals and starved of organic matter. As a result, vegetation is deprived of basic nutrients.

An important part of Scheussler's theory is that any deficiency of a mineral salt will impair the cells' ability to assimilate and utilize the organic compounds that they require. Apart from some acute conditions in the early stages of disease, it has been found that the salts work more effectively when two or more are combined. Thanks to the research of Dr Maurice Blackmore and Dr Leslie H. Fisher, we now know that:

- Mineral deficiencies are the common denominator of most illnesses.

- Mineral deficiencies very rarely exist singly.

- Most chronic conditions are the result of at least three and often as many as six mineral deficiencies.

- Each of these mineral salts acts uniquely. Contrary to standard biochemistry, a deficiency in them cannot be

Tissue salt	General indications	Indications on iris, pupil and tongue	Symptom qualifications: < = makes patient worse > = makes patient better	Summary of action
Calc fluor (calcium fluoride)	Over-relaxed tissue (prolapses)	Cracked tongue	<Damp, changeable weather >Heat and warm applications	Tissue strengthener
Calc phos (calcium phosphate)	Malnourished muscles, bone or blood; frequent infections in children	Poor texture of iris	<Cold and wet >Warm and dry	Cell builder
Calc sulph (calcium sulphate)	Reproductive organs, hay fever, skin problems	Inflamed eyes with thick yellow discharge; flabby tongue with yellow coating	—	General cleanser
Ferr phos (iron phosphate)	Acute inflammation; tiredness and pallor	Red tongue	<Heat; excitement; jarring movements >Cold applications; rest	Inflammation remover
Kali mur (potassium chloride)	Glandular swellings; white, sticky mucus	White or greyish fur on tongue	<Rich, fatty food; morning; seaside >Cold applications	Congestion remover

Remedy	Conditions	Signs	Worse (<) / Better (>)	Function
Kali phos (potassium phosphate)	Lowered nervous energy	White or greyish-white fur on tongue; dilated pupils	<Worry; mental exertion >Company; eating	Nerve power activator
Kali sulph (potassium sulphate)	Skin problems	White spots on outer part of iris	<Hot, stuffy room; late afternoon >Cool, fresh air	Cell oxygenator
Mag phos (magnesium phosphate)	Tremors; nerve pain; insomnia; confusion	Pupils constricted or misshapen	<Cold, alcohol >Warmth; bending double	Nerve and muscle fibre nutrient
Nat phos (sodium phosphate)	Acidity; indigestion	Creamy fur at back of tongue	<Afternoon; open air >Warmth	Acid neutralizer
Nat mur (sodium chloride)	Shock, bad circulation, cramp, palpitations, migraine, arthritic and rheumatic pain, suppressed emotions	Sodium ring around iris, deep-cracked tongue	<Noise, warm room, seaside, at 10.00a.m., lying down >Cold bath, open air, lying on right side, tight clothing	Good for blood circulation and general aches and pains
Nat sulph (sodium sulphate)	Water retention	No fur on tongue, or greyish-brown at base	<Hot, humid or damp weather >Dry warmth	Remover of excess fluid
Silicea (silica)	All chronic conditions, especially arthritis	—	<Cold, dry air	Remover of excess calcium

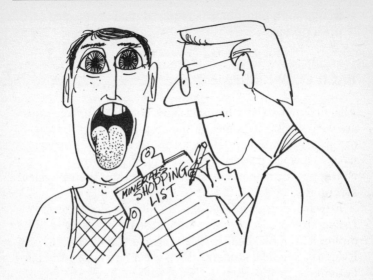

THE IRIS, PUPIL AND TONGUE CAN FURNISH IMPORTANT INFORMATION ABOUT MINERAL DEFICIENCY...

overcome even if the metal and the salt are present in other combinations. For example, even though sodium chloride and potassium phosphate may be present in adequate quantities, this will not make up for a deficiency of sodium phosphate or potassium chloride. Dr Paul Cullinan, an Australian biochemist, recently carried out a great deal of research to establish the validity of this hypothesis.

- Symptoms are of primary importance as indicators of mineral deficiencies. In particular, the iris, pupil and tongue can furnish important information when taken in conjunction with other symptoms and signs.

- Normally a metal is required only once in a prescription.

- A sodium salt is required in every prescription.

- Two sulphates should not appear in the same prescription.

- Magnesium phosphate is required in almost every prescription.

BACH FLOWER REMEDIES

Although not strictly homeopathic, Bach flower remedies are very similar to homeopathic preparations in that they are greatly diluted and do not work on a purely physical basis. They are prescribed according to patients' characters and emotional states rather than their physical symptoms.

Edward Bach, a Welshman, qualified as a doctor at University College, London and subsequently gained his diploma in public health at Cambridge University in 1913. Even as a medical student, Bach was more interested in patients as people than in their diseases. In particular, he noted that certain patients recovered more quickly than others, and he found that these were invariably the ones who were happy, emotionally healthy and positive thinkers. On the other hand, those who were full of 'negative' emotions, such as anxiety and worry, and who

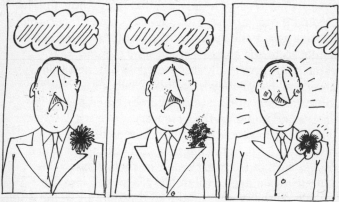

BACH... ASSIDUOUSLY SEARCHED FOR THE PLANTS WHICH WOULD REVERSE THE EFFECTS OF NEGATIVE THINKING...

lacked hope and cheerfulness recovered much more slowly.

Bach came to the conclusion that the body is the mirror of the soul, and reflected its mental or emotional condition. He decided that the real basis of disease was in the mind and spirit, and that in order to recover physically, patients needed help to overcome negative emotions. He became very impressed with the concepts of homeopathy, which held that the patient rather than the disease was of paramount importance.

Bach spent a number of years working at the Royal London Homeopathic Hospital, and noted that patients with the same emotional states tended to need the same remedy. He began to prescribe on the basis of his patients' mental temperaments and was extremely successful. Then in 1930, at the peak of his career, Bach abandoned his medical practice in order to follow an instinctual feeling that the solution to illness could be found in trees and plants.

He left London for the countryside, where he began his research. He developed an extreme sensitivity that enabled him to communicate with plants and experience in himself their various qualities. For the next seven years, he assiduously searched for the plants which would reverse the effects of negative thinking. It seems that he adopted the negative emotional states himself, and when he came across the appropriate plant for that particular mental state, his normal serene state of mind was restored. He eventually discovered 38 different wild flowers, all completely harmless, which would heal the unfortunate mental states that predisposed people to disease and impaired their recovery.

Bach began preparing his flower remedies by picking the blooms early in the morning and placing them in a glass bowl of pure spring water; he then exposed the contents to sunlight until midday. The action of the sunlight on the flowers produced tiny bubbles in the water, which he then decanted, bottled and preserved with a little alcohol. Early blossoms (mostly from trees) were covered

with water in sterile containers as soon as possible; these
were then boiled gently for half an hour and the flowers
removed after cooling. The liquid was then filtered and
bottled, with a little added alcohol as a preservative.

The Bach flower remedies
These are classified into seven groups according to the
relevant predominant emotion.

Fear

Aspen	Vague fears that something terrible will happen.
Cherry plum	Fear of doing something impulsive and immoral.
Mimulus	Fear of poverty and misfortune.
Red chestnut	Fear for others.
Rock rose	Fear with no hope.

Despondency

Crab apple	Unclean feelings. House-proud.
Elm	Temporary inadequacy.
Larch	Expectations of failure; lack of confidence.
Oak	Brave determination of 'plodding' type.
Pine	Lack of self-respect; guilt feelings.
Star of Bethlehem	Shock from bad news.
Sweet chestnut	Absolute dejection.
Willow	Resentment and bitterness.

Uncertainty

Cerato	Doubt of own judgement.
Gentian	Easy discouragement.
Gorse	Pessimism and defeatism.
Hornbeam	Procrastination.
Scleranthus	Indecision; fluctuating moods.
Wild oat	Lack of knowledge of intended path in life.

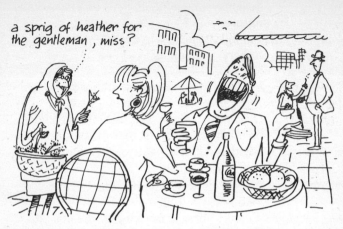

HEATHER FOR TALKATIVE SELF-CENTRED BORES....

Lack of interest

Chestnut bud	Inability to learn by experience.
Clematis	Indifference, absent-mindedness and dreaminess.
Honeysuckle	Nostalgia and homesickness.
Mustard	Sudden feeling that a 'dark cloud' has descended.
Olive	Energy-drained.
White chestnut	Persistent unwanted thoughts.
Wild rose	Drifting without ambition; apathy.

Loneliness

Heather	Talkativeness; self-centredness; a bore.
Impatiens	Impatience and irritability.
Water violet	Pride; reserved, sometimes superior nature.

Over-sensitivity to influence and ideas

Agrimony	Inner torture with facade of cheerfulness.
Centaury	Inability to say no; 'human doormat'.

Holly	Jealousy; vengeful, envious and suspicious nature.
Walnut	Inability to adjust to change — for example, puberty, menopause.

Excessive care for the welfare of others

Beech	Arrogance and criticism of others.
Chicory	Over-possessiveness, a martyr; insistence on others conforming to own standards.
Rock water	Rigid in outlook; overly high standards for self.
Vervain	Fanaticism; incensed by injustice.
Vine	Domination, inflexibility and ambition.

In acute mental conditions, these flower remedies are known to have brought relief almost instantly. In chronic mental conditions, they have to be taken regularly for a longer period. Nevertheless, they can have quite a dramatic influence on improving a patient's general attitude and therefore helping with physical recovery.

Unlike most homeopathic medicines, Bach flower remedies may be taken regularly and with or without food. Place a few drops of the chosen remedy or remedies into a glass of water (the bottles containing the remedies come complete with special droppers to make this easier) and sip this slowly; if no water is available, hold a few drops in the mouth for a few seconds, and then swallow. The remedies should be taken three times per day for at least several months, even if some improvement is noted straight away.

Rescue remedy

This is used for shock and trauma (physical or mental). 'Rescue remedy' is a combination of five flowers — cherry plum, clematis, impatiens, rock rose and star of Bethlehem — and is used in an emergency when people receive bad news, become severely upset and/or experience something startling, including accidents that affect the mind. Rescue remedy may be applied as a

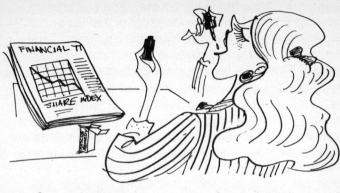

RESCUE REMEDY : FOR ANY SHOCK ...

cream to a particular area or taken by mouth by adding four drops to a little water. Continue the medication every one to four hours until symptoms are relieved.

HOMEOPUNCTURE

This is the judicious combination of two types of treatment: acupuncture and homeopathy. An acupuncture needle is dipped into the selected homeopathic remedy and then placed in the relevant acupuncture point. Apart from the obvious advantage of receiving two treatments for the price of one, each therapy is more effective than it would be if used on its own. In addition, the precautions that need to be taken during homeopathic treatment in terms of food, drink, scented products and so on (see pages 37-8) are unnecessary with homeopuncture as the remedies go straight to the relevant part of the body.

COMPLEX HOMEOPATHY

This system, like classical homeopathy, originated in Germany and has been in use for a considerable time. Complex homeopathy consists of prescribing mixtures of homeopathic remedies in low potency, and carefully preparing these combinations in order to provide a comprehensive treatment for a specific condition. Prescribing, therefore, is based upon particular (named) diseases. This is not because complex homeopathy necessarily recognizes the individual existence of such diseases, but merely because their names represent specific clusters of symptoms which can be covered by particular remedies. In fact, there may be several complex remedies for any one named disease according to the way in which it manifests itself in an individual.

For example, one pharmacy produces seven complex remedies for the relatively simple condition *cystitis* (inflammation of the bladder):

	Complex remedy	Indications for use
1	*Uva ursi* oplx (complex)	Especially for those who also suffer from rheumatism
2	*Echinacea ang* oplx	Anti-inflammatory and booster
3	*Juniperus* oplx	Kidney involvement
4	*Natrium carb* oplx	Gouty disposition
5	*Millefolium* oplx	Blood in the urine
6	*Acid benzioc* oplx	Offensive-smelling urine
7	*Climicifuga* oplx	Acute cystitis during menopause

Now let us look in detail at the formulae of the first two remedies. First, here are the constituents (and their potencies) and indications/actions of *uva ursi* oplx:

Constituents	Indications/Actions
Uva ursi 2x	Frequent passing of water
Cannabis sativa 3x	Irritation of urinary tract
Clematis recta 3x	Sensitivity to cold
Hypericum perforatum 1x	Irritability of nerves

Plantago major 1x	Frequent passing of water
Rhus aromatica 5x	Difficulty in passing water

Compare this with *echinacea ang* oplx:

Constituents	**Indications/Actions**
Echinacea ang 2x	General lack of resistance
Arctium lappa 4x	Infection of mucous membranes
Baptisia tinctoria 2x	Intestinal symptoms
Colocynthis 4x	Irritation of peritoneum
Lachesis 8x	General raised sensitivity
Rhus toxicodendron 6x	Infection
Mercurius cyanatus 4x	Inflammation of mucous membranes; removal of toxins
Sulphur 6x	Sluggish response to infection

Clearly, no disease is straightforward, nor are the remedies used in complex homeopathy.

PENDULUMS

Some homeopathic practitioners use pendulums to help them to select remedies. To the uninitiated, this technique may seem strange, but it is centuries old, having been used by the ancients not only to reveal the most appropriate remedies, but also to discover water, among many other things.

Swinging a pendulum is simply one way in which a person can contact his or her own innate intelligence, or subconscious. Its use presupposes that the practitioner's subconscious mind already knows the correct remedy. This knowledge is often thought to be drawn from a universal intelligence, and the use of the pendulum is one way of tapping it.

APPLIED KINESIOLOGY

This is a relatively modern approach that employs muscle testing to find out what the body requires. Although some recent criticism has called this method into question, it does seem to have a degree of validity. It works by observing that one of a patient's arm muscles is strengthened when a correct remedy is placed in the mouth or near the lips or held in his or her hand.

The biggest problem in kinesiology is that there may be two remedies that effectively strengthen the muscle, but the one that causes the muscle to have the greater resistance when locked is the indicated remedy. This test can also be used to identify foods to which a patient may be allergic or in which he or she may be deficient.

BIOENERGETIC MEDICINE

This is a form of medicine that employs a variety of sophisticated instruments to test the electrical potential of various points on the body. The work was started by Reinhard Voll, who not only plotted areas of low resistance and found them to coincide with the known acupuncture points, but also found others that he described as 'reference' points to all parts of the body. By measuring one of these, it is possible to detect any abnormality that may exist in the part of the body to which it relates.

When a measurement is abnormal, a correction may be brought about by a number of treatments, including classical and complex homeopathic remedies. In addition, preparations from various body tissues are also employed. These are primarily taken from glands such as the pituitary, thyroid, ovaries, adrenals and thymus. However, tissue from any part of the body may be prepared in a homeopathic potency and used specifically for problems in that area. These remedies are sometimes called *sarcoids*.

ISOPATHY

Isopathy differs from homeopathy in that it treats diseases or conditions with the substances that actually cause them — it involves treating 'same with same', not (as in homeopathy) 'like with like'. For example, hayfever sufferers are given a potency of pollen, and those allergic to cat fur, housedust, mites or certain foods are given potencies of these substances. Sometimes the patient's own diseased tissue is used to make a remedy.

Isopathy, then, is similar to the immunizations used in orthodox medicine, when a weakened strain of a micro-organism is given to cause the body to build up an immunity to a particular disease. In isopathy, however, the homeopathic dilutions used are, of course, very much weaker. Some homeopaths who use this system obtain remarkable results, especially when it is combined with conventional homeopathy.

FURTHER READING

Anderson, David, Buegel, Dale & Chernin, Dennis, *Homoeopathic Remedies for Physicians, Laymen and Therapists*, Himalayan International Institute, 1978.

Bach, Edward, *Heal Thyself: An Explanation of the Real Cause and Cure of Disease*, C.W. Daniel, 1931.

Batra, Mukesh, *Homoeopathy: Everyman's Guide to Natural Health*, Mayfair Paperback/Arnold-Heinemann (India), 1982.

Carey, George W. & Perry, Edward L., *The Biochemical System of Medicine*, Haren & Brother (Calcutta), 1971.

Clover, Ann, *Homeopathy, A Patient's Guide*, Thorsons, 1984.

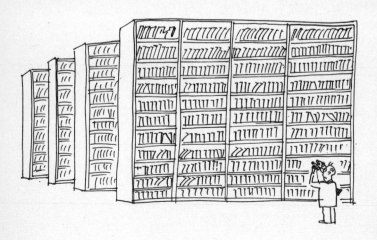

Chitkara, H.C., *Speaking of Homoeopathy*, Oriental UP, 1987.

Gibson, D.M., *First Aid Homoeopathy in Accidents and Ailments*, British Homeopathic Association, 1986.

Ross, Gordon, *Homoeopathy: An Introductory Guide*, Thorsons, 1976.

Sheppherd, Dorothy, *Homoeopathy in Epidemic Diseases*, Health Science Press, 1967.

——, *Homoeopathy for the First-Aider*, Health Science Press, 1972.

Sheppard, K., *Treatment of Cats by Homoeopathy*, C.W. Daniels, 1963.

——, *Treatment of Dogs by Homoeopathy*, C.W. Daniels, 1967.

Singh, Yudhvir, *Homeopathic Cure for Common Diseases*, Orient Publications, 1979.

Speight, Leslie J., *Homoeopathy and Immunisation*, Health Science Press, 1983.

——, *Homoeopathy: A Practical Guide to Natural Medicine*, Granada, 1979.

——, *Homoeopathy for Emergencies*, C.W. Daniel, 1984, Vithoulkas, George, *Homoeopathy: Medicine of the New Man*, Thorsons, 1979.

Weiner, Michael & Goss, Kathleen, *The Complete Book of Homeopathy*, Bantam, 1982.

USEFUL ADDRESSES

ASSOCIATIONS AND SOCIETIES

Britain
Association of Natural Medicines
27 Braintree Road
Witham
Essex CM8 2DD
Tel: (0376) 511069

British Homoeopathic Association
27a Devonshire Street
London W1N 1RJ
Tel: (01) 935 2163

Society of Homoeopaths
16 St Michael's Mount
Northampton NN1 4JG
Tel: (0604) 28767

Hahnemann Society
Humane Education Centre
Avenue Lodge
Bounds Green Road
London N22 4EU
Tel: (01) 889 1595

New Zealand
New Zealand Homoeopathic Society
P O 2939
Auckland

United States
American Foundation for Homeopathy
1508 S. Garfield
Alhambra
California 91801

American Institute of Homeopathy
Suite 41
1500 Massachusetts Ave NW
Washington, DC 20005
Tel: (202) 223-6182

International Foundation for Homeopathy
2366 Eastlake Avenue E301
Seattle
Washington 98102

National Center for Homeopathy
Suite 506
6231 Leesburg Pike
Falls Church
Virginia 22044

HOMEOPATHIC HOSPITALS AND PRACTITIONERS

Britain
Although homeopathic treatment is included under the NHS, you must specify that you wish to be referred to a homeopathic physician — otherwise, treatment will be given along orthodox lines.

Bristol Homeopathic Hospital
St Michael's Hill
Cotham
Bristol BS6 6JU
Tel: (0272) 731231

Glasgow Homeopathic Hospital
1000 Great Western Road
Glasgow G12 0NR
Tel: (041) 339 0382

Glasgow Homeopathic Out-Patients Dept
5 Lynedoch Crescent
Glasgow G3 6EQ
Tel: (041) 332 4490

The Homeopathic Hospital
Church Road
Tunbridge Wells
Kent TN1 1JU
Tel: (0892) 42977

Mossley Hill Hospital
Park Avenue
Aigburth
Liverpool L18 8BT
Tel: (051) 724 2335

Royal London Homeopathic Hospital
Great Ormond Street
London WC1N 3HR
Tel: (01) 837 8833

To find a homeopathic practitioner, contact the British
Homeopathic Association (for medically qualified
homeopathic doctors in the UK and abroad, as well as
dentists, veterinarians, pharmacists and manufacturers)
or the Society of Homeopaths (qv). The quarterly journal
Homeopathy Today (available from the Hahnemann
Society) lists clinics where private treatment can be
obtained from medically qualified homeopathic doctors

Argentina
Homeopathic Centre
Juncal 2884
1425 Buenos Aires
Tel: (01) 821 2911

Australia
Australian Institute of Homeopathy
21 Bulah Close
Berowra Heights
Sydney, NSW 2082

Canada
Canadian College of Natural Healing
380 Forest Street
Ottawa
Ontario K2B 8E6

Greece
Medical Institute for Homeopathic Research and
Application
c/o Dr Spiro Diamantides
20 Dragoumi Str.
CR-115 28 Athens

India
Bengal Allen Medical Institute
169/B Bowbazar Street
Calcutta 700 012

Jai Khodiyar Cosmic Healing Centre
25 Yojana
Tilak Nagar
Bombay 400 004
Tel: 387601

New Zealand
Homeopathic & Naturopathic Centre
c/o Dr Thomas J. Baker
22 Cockayne Road
Ngaio
Wellington
Tel: 04-843-427/04-857-440

Singapore
Justin Morais
73 Bloxhome Drive
Singapore
Tel: 2880271

Sri Lanka
Medicina Alternativa
28 International Buddhist Centre Road
Colombo 6

United States
Health Consciousness
Shangri-la Lane
PO Box 550
Oviedo
Florida 32765-0550

Hom Boeriche & Tafel
Homeopathic Healthcare
1011 Arch Street
Philadelphia
Pennsylvania 19107
Tel: (215) 922-2967

American Institute of Homeopathy
Suite 41
1500 Massachusetts Ave NW
Washington, DC 20005
Tel: (202) 223-6182

SUPPLIERS

Homeopathic remedies

Britain
Ainsworths
38 New Cavendish Street
London W1M 7LH
Tel: (01) 935 5330

Buxton & Grant
176 Whiteladies Road
Bristol BS8 2XU
Tel: (0272) 735025

Fossway
38 Harepath Road
Seaton
Devon EX12 2RU
Tel: (0297) 20414

Galen Pharmacy
1 South Terrace
 South Street
Dorchester
Dorset
Tel: (0305) 63996

E. Gould & Son Ltd
14 Crowndale Road
London NW1 1TT
Tel: (01) 388 4752

House of Mistry
15-17 South End Road
Hampstead Heath
London NW3
Tel: (01) 794 0848

Hughes' Chemist
High Street
High Wycombe
Bucks
Tel: (0494) 30138

Neal's Yard Apothecary
2 Neal's Yard
Covent Garden
London WC2
Tel: (01) 379 7222

Nelson Pharmacies Ltd
73 Duke Street
Grosvenor Square
London W1M 6BY
Tel: (01) 629 3118

Weleda (UK) Ltd
Heanor Road
Ilkeston
Derbyshire DE7 8DR
Tel: (0602) 303151

United States

Boiron/Borneman
1208 Amosland Road
Norwood
Pennsylvania 19074

Homeopathic Medicines
6125 W. Tropicana Avenue
Las Vegas
Nevada 89103

Standard Homeopathic Co.
PO Box 61067
Los Angeles
California 90061

Bach flower remedies

Australia
Nonesuch Botanical Pty Ltd
PO Box 68
Mount Evelyn
Victoria 3796
Tel: (03) 762 8577

Britain
Dr Edward Bach Centre
Mount Vernon
Sotwell
Wallingford
Oxon OX10 0PZ

United States
Ellpon (Bach USA) Inc.
PO Box 320
Woodmere
New York 11598

ABOUT THE AUTHOR

Dr Nelson Brunton was educated in India, Sri Lanka and England, and qualified as a doctor in Sri Lanka.

He is an experienced practitioner of natural therapies – acupuncture, naturopathy as well as homeopathy. He lectures on these subjects around the world, and is Visiting Professor for Medicina Alternativa.

Dr Brunton writes for *Natural Medicine* and this is his third book.

MEDITATION

Erica Smith and Nicholas Wilks

Meditation is a state of inner stillness which has been cultivated by mystics for thousands of years. The main reason for its recent popularity is that regular practice has been found to improve mental and physical health, largely due to its role in alleviating stress.

price £5.99

HYPNOSIS

Ursula Markham

Hypnosis has a remarkable record of curing a wide range of ills. Ursula Markham, a practising hypnotherapist, explains how, by releasing inner tensions, hypnosis can help people to heal themselves.

price £5.99

AROMATHERAPY

Gill Martin

Aromatherapy uses the essential oils of plants, which are massaged into the skin, added to baths or taken internally to treat a variety of ailments and enhance general well-being.

price £5.99

ENCYCLOPAEDIA OF NATURAL MEDICINE

Michael Murray and Joseph Pizzorno

The Encyclopaedia of Natural Medicine is the most comprehensive guide and reference to the use of natural measures in the maintenance of good health and the prevention and treatment of disease. It explains the principles of natural medicine and outlines their application through the safe and effective use of herbs, vitamins, minerals, diet and nutritional supplements, and covers an extensive range of health conditions, from asthma to depression, from psoriasis to candidiasis, from diabetes to the common cold.

price £13.99

ISBN 0-356-17218 X

ACUPUNCTURE
Dr Michael Nightingale

Acupuncture is a traditional Chinese therapy which usually (but not always) uses needles to stimulate the body's own energy and so bring healing. The author is a practising acupuncturist well aware of the particular concerns of first-time patients.

price £5.99

ALEXANDER TECHNIQUE
Chris Stevens

Alexander Technique is a way of becoming more aware of balance, posture and movement in everyday activities. It can not only cure various complaints related to posture, such as backache, but teaches people to use their body more effectively and reduces stress.

price £5.99

All Optima books are available at your bookshop or newsagent, or can be ordered from the following address:
Little, Brown and Company (UK) Limited,
P.O. Box 11,
Falmouth,
Cornwall TR10 9EN.

Alternatively you may fax your order to the above address. Fax No. 0326 376423.

Payments can be made as follows: cheque, postal order (payable to Little, Brown and Company) or by credit cards, Visa/Access. Do not send cash or currency. UK customers and B.F.P.O. please allow £1.00 for postage and packing for the first book, plus 50p for the second book, plus 30p for each additional book up to a maximum charge of £3.00 (7 books plus).

Overseas customers including Ireland, please allow £2.00 for the first book plus £1.00 for the second book, plus 50p for each additional book.

NAME (Block Letters) ....

....

ADDRESS ....

....

....

☐ I enclose my remittance for _____

☐ I wish to pay by Access/Visa Card

Number ☐☐☐☐☐☐☐☐☐☐☐☐☐☐☐☐

Card Expiry Date ☐☐☐☐